THE

Back

BOOK

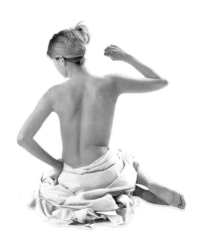

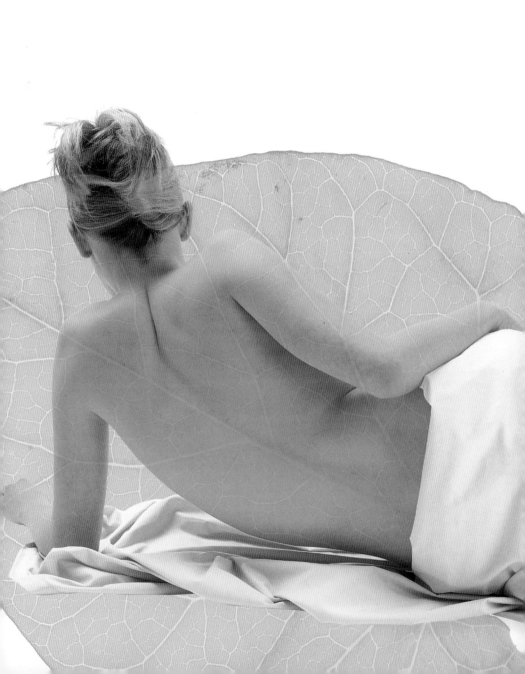

THE
Back
BOOK

JANE HOBDEN & SUE TUCKER
Consulting osteopath: DEBORAH DOOLE

APPLE

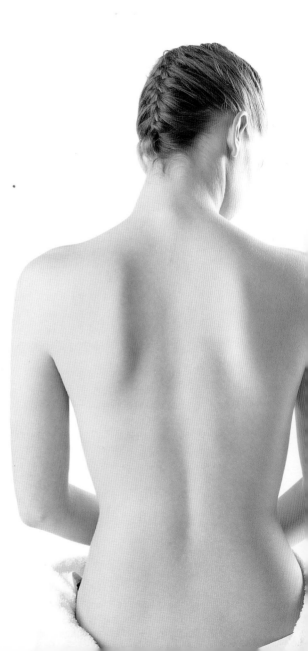

A QUARTO BOOK

Published by
Apple Press
The Old Brewery
6 Blundell Street
London N7 9BH

ISBN: 1 84092 224 9

QUAR.BKPK

Conceived, designed, and produced by
Quarto Publishing plc
The Old Brewery
6 Blundell Street
London N7 9BH

Editor: Michelle Pickering
Art editor: Sally Bond
Assistant art director: Penny Cobb
Designer: Sheila Volpe
Photographers: Paola Zucchi, Colin Bowling
Illustrator: Peter Campbell
Indexer: Dorothy Frame

Art director: Moira Clinch
Publisher: Piers Spence

Manufactured by Regent Publishing Services Ltd,
Hong Kong
Printed by Leefung-Asco Printers Ltd, China

TO THE READER

This book is not a medical reference book. The
advice it contains is general, not specific, and
neither the authors, the consulting osteopath, nor
the publisher can be held responsible for any
adverse reactions to the recipes, techniques, and
suggestions contained herein. Any application of
the recipes, techniques, and suggestions is at the
reader's sole discretion and risk.

contents

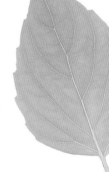

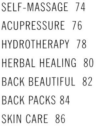

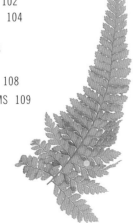

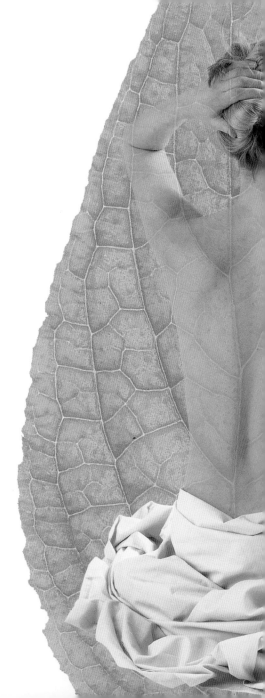

Introduction

Like the skeleton in a leaf, the spine provides the back with support and flexibility. Having a strong, healthy back is central to our physical well-being, and is often taken for granted by those who are fortunate enough to have one. Yet almost a third of adults suffer from back problems each year. You don't have to be one of them – just follow the advice in this book to keep your back in good working order.

First, you need to know how your back works to understand why things can go wrong. Then you need to think about how you use your back; so many back problems are caused by poor posture, or by carrying out everyday activities in ways that strain the back. This book explains how to make simple postural and lifestyle changes that will help to prevent this type of backache.

A healthy back is a strong and supple back. The book contains a series of easy-to-follow, step-by-step exercises, specially designed by an osteopath to develop your back's strength and suppleness and so reduce the risk of injury or strain.

Another element of back health is relaxation. Massage, aromatherapy, and hydrotherapy are enjoyable ways of relaxing at any time, but they are especially beneficial when you have an aching back.

Remember, too, that backs need pampering just as much as the rest of our bodies. Make back care part of your regular beauty routine and you'll keep your back looking and feeling good. Try the back pack recipes for a smoother, softer, more beautiful back.

Finally, there is information on what you can do about acute or persistent back problems if they do occur. A range of complementary therapies is described, and a series of exercises is outlined for specific back ailments.

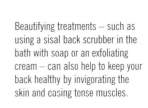

Beautifying treatments – such as using a sisal back scrubber in the bath with soap or an exfoliating cream – can also help to keep your back healthy by invigorating the skin and easing tense muscles.

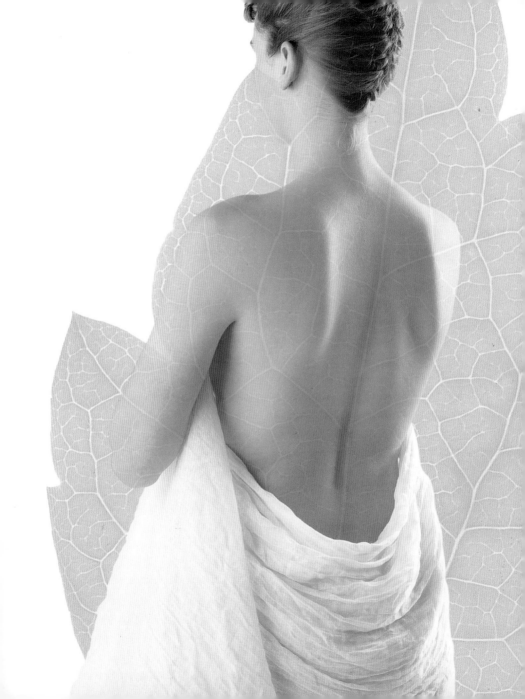

Looking after your Back

THIS CHAPTER LOOKS AT HOW THE BACK WORKS AND OFFERS ADVICE ON POSTURE. THERE IS ALSO GUIDANCE ON TACKLING DAY-TO-DAY ACTIVITIES, SUCH AS HOUSEWORK, GARDENING, AND SHOPPING, IN A BACK-FRIENDLY WAY. FINALLY, THERE IS A STEP-BY-STEP STRETCHING ROUTINE TO HELP KEEP YOUR BACK STRONG AND SUPPLE.

HOW THE **BACK WORKS**

The back, with its central column of bones and cartilage – the spine – is a hugely complex part of the human anatomy. The spine extends from the base of the skull to the tailbone, and curves in three places – at neck, chest, and lower back level. This makes the spine flexible and creates a concertina effect, which is better for absorbing shocks and stresses. The spine has three main functions: to support the human skeleton, to protect the spinal cord, and to help us move freely.

The vertebrae

The spine is made up of 33 interlocking bones, known as vertebrae. Of these, 24 are mobile and the rest are permanently fused. Each of the mobile vertebrae is connected to the next by a joint, known as a facet joint, which stabilizes the spinal column and allows it to move appropriately – the cervical and lumbar facets are designed for easy movement, the thoracic facets for restricted movement in order to hold the ribcage in place.

THE VERTEBRAE

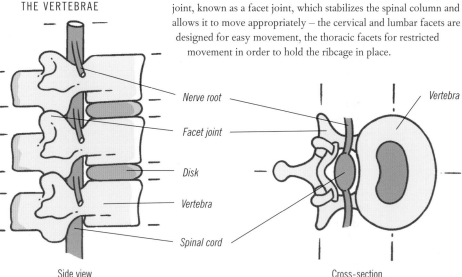

Nerve root

Facet joint

Disk

Vertebra

Spinal cord

Vertebra

Side view

Cross-section

Sacrum and coccyx

At the base of the 24 mobile vertebrae are the sacrum and coccyx. The sacrum is a flat triangular bone formed by five fused sacral vertebrae; the coccyx – often known as the tailbone – lies below the sacrum and is formed from four fused coccygeal vertebrae.

Disks

The 24 mobile vertebrae are separated from each other by disks, thick pads of cartilage that are wedged between each pair of vertebrae to act as shock absorbers. Inside each disk is a soft gel. During daily activities, the water content of the disk is diminished through compression; the disks are rehydrated at night when we lie down and rest. This is the reason why we are taller in the mornings than in the evenings.

The spinal cord

On the outer side of each of the 24 mobile vertebrae is a bony arch – these arches are the knobbles you feel when you run your fingers down your spine. Inside the arches lies the spinal canal, through which the spinal cord runs. The spinal cord contains bundles of nerves and is effectively an extension of the brain.

Muscles

Many different muscles support the spine. Deep muscles running parallel to the spine – the paraspinal muscles – keep it upright; muscles in the pelvis – the abdominal, buttock, and thigh muscles – influence its position, affecting the lumbar curve at the small of the back.

THE SPINE

Cervical curve
(7 cervical vertebrae)

Thoracic curve
(12 thoracic vertebrae)

Paraspinal muscles

Lumbar curve
(5 lumbar vertebrae)

The sacrum, and below it, the coccyx

POSTURE **MATTERS**

Good posture is the key to a healthy back. A good posture is one that enables the skeleton to hold itself upright and to carry itself most effectively. Poor posture strains the skeleton, causes pain, and can eventually lead to a bent and stooped back. With a little practice, you will be able to recognize and correct poor habits in your posture. Children should be shown how to sit and stand properly from an early age – this will help them to avoid poor posture as they get older.

Sitting pretty

Most of us spend a lot of time sitting down, so it is important to make sure that our backs are properly supported when seated. Always make sure that your hips are pushed against the back of the chair and that the chair gives your lower back adequate support. Try to sit straight with your feet flat on the floor; avoid slouching or crossing your legs. When lounging in easy chairs, avoid sitting in a slumped or twisted position – however comfortable it may seem! – because this can eventually lead to back stiffness and pain. When you are sitting for any length of time, get up and move about regularly – this will help to keep your muscle tone, joints, and circulation healthy.

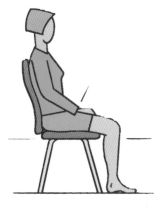

Good sitting posture
The ideal chair is one in which you can sit upright, with your hips against the back of the seat and both feet flat on the floor.

Good standing posture

Stand tall and relaxed. Lift the top of your head, keep your chin tucked in, and hold your shoulders back. Imagine a string running through the center of your body from your feet to your head, pulling you up straight.

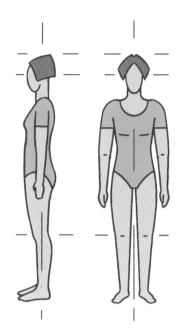

Standing straight

Standing properly not only helps to keep the back healthy, it can also have a powerful effect on your sense of well-being. When standing, avoid rounding your back and slouching. Imagine a thread running through the center of your body from the top of your head to the base of your feet, and that you are being lifted up by the thread. Practice standing like this. The aim is to stand easily, using minimal effort; eventually, this way of standing will become automatic. When standing for long periods, try to maintain good posture and move your legs around regularly to prevent circulation problems.

Walking tall

Maintaining a good posture when standing will ensure that you walk properly, too. Walk tall and stay relaxed, with your head up and shoulders back. Let your arms swing freely. If you are walking any distance, choose shoes with a moderate heel. Avoid high-heeled shoes, which force the pelvis to tilt forward, causing the lower back to arch excessively.

Lifting

When lifting something heavy, keep your back straight and your weight equally distributed on both feet. Stand close to the item you wish to lift and squat rather than bend at the waist. As you straighten up, let your leg muscles do the work. Do not try to lift heavy loads just because you think you should be able to – be aware of what you can realistically manage.

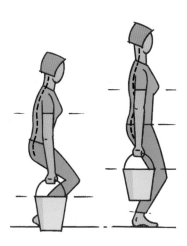

Lifting a heavy object
When lifting a load, squat rather than stoop, then straighten up, letting your legs bear the weight. Keep your back as straight as possible throughout.

Lying on your side
The most comfortable position when lying on your side is with the back straight but relaxed, and the knees drawn up and bent at right angles to the body.

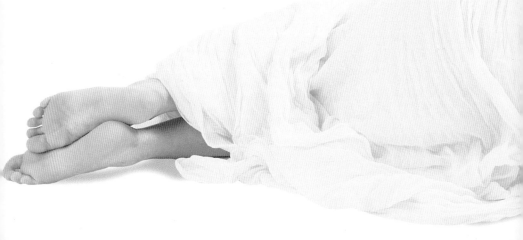

Carrying

Carrying heavy loads in the hands and arms, on the shoulders, or on the back can put a lot of stress on the joints of the spine. If you are carrying two loads, such as two bags of shopping, make sure that the weight is evenly distributed. When carrying luggage, it is far better for your back if you use two small suitcases rather than a single large one.

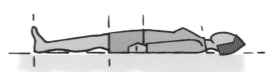

Lying down

Lying down in a way that enables your back to relax fully is another important element of good posture. When lying down, the spine is relieved of the pressure of bearing weight, so enjoy stretching out your body in this relaxed situation. Always go to sleep in a comfortable position, but bear in mind that most of us adopt many different positions during sleep. For most people, lying face down feels uncomfortable and can cause neck strain.

Lying on your back

Lie on your back on a supportive surface, such as a firm mattress or a rug on the floor. Stretch your legs out and hold your arms loosely across your body or at your sides. For maximum relaxation, you may feel more comfortable if you raise your feet slightly with a pillow.

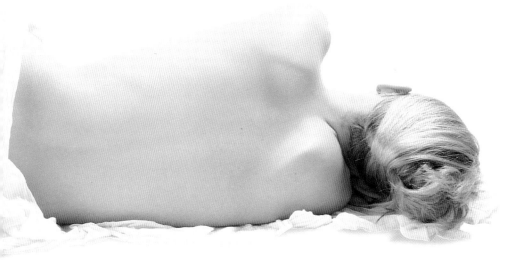

EVERYDAY **ACTIVITIES**

Everyday activities, both inside and outside the home, are full of potential pitfalls for our backs. Housework, lifting and carrying babies and children, driving, shopping, and gardening all involve bending and twisting the spine, and increasing the weight burden on our backs. It is important that we are aware of the potential risks involved in these activities and learn the safe way to do them.

Housework

Most household tasks can strain the back. Pushing a vacuum cleaner, moving furniture, ironing, cleaning the bathtub, and sweeping the kitchen floor are all activities that involve twisting and bending the spine. When cleaning the bathtub, kneel close to it so that you can reach inside without having to bend over and stretch down. Make sure items such as vacuum cleaners, brooms, and ironing boards are the right height for you, so that you can use them comfortably without having to bend over them. When an activity involves bending repeatedly, try not to do too much at once and stop regularly to stretch.

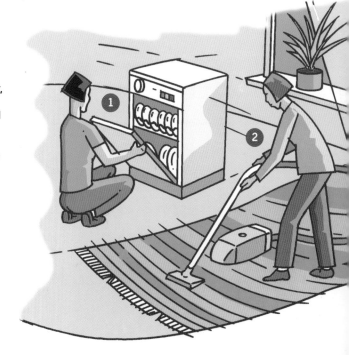

1 **Low kitchen fittings**
If kitchen cupboards and fittings, such as ovens and dishwashers, are situated at floor level, always squat in front of them, keeping your back straight, rather than stoop from the waist.

2 **Vacuuming** This involves bending repeatedly, so vacuum the house in short sessions rather than all at once, and intersperse vacuuming with other activities, such as dusting, to counteract the bending movements. Stop regularly to stretch.

Carrying children

Lifting and moving small children around can be a major source of backache. Choose a crib with a drop-down side so that you do not have to pick up the baby at arm's length. When the baby is small, she or he can be strapped into a carrier in front of you so that the weight is supported by your abdomen and chest. When the baby grows bigger, use a carrier strapped to your back. As soon as the baby can sit up independently, use a buggy.

3 **Picking up toddlers** Squat down to their level and lift them up close to you, but avoid carrying them for any distance. If you have to hold a child for any length of time, swap sides regularly.

4 **Harnesses** These are a back-friendly way of carrying babies. Strap small babies to your front, bigger ones to your back.

5 **Cribs** Choose a crib with a drop-down side so that you do not strain your back by bending over the side of the crib and picking up the baby at arm's length.

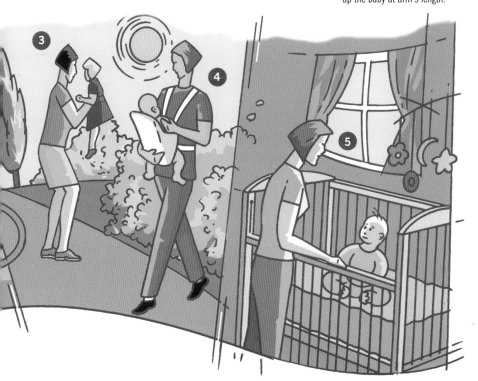

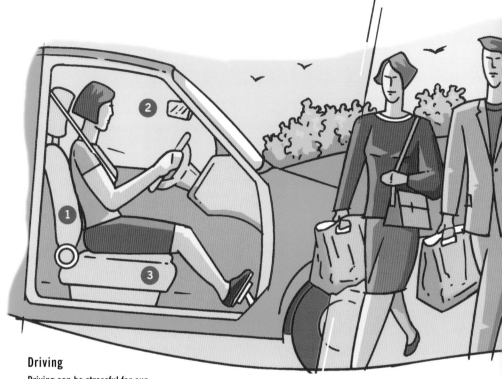

Driving

Driving can be stressful for our backs. Ideally, car seats should offer the same kind of support as a firm chair. Your back should be straight or slightly reclining, with your spine supported up to your head, and your hips roughly parallel with your knees. Adjust the seat to give your back maximum support and to allow you to reach the pedals comfortably. Also make sure that the headrest lies close to the back of your head. You should be able to reach the steering wheel without overstretching, with your arms slightly bent at the elbows.

1 **Car seat** It should support your whole spine, and you should be able to reach the pedals and the steering wheel easily without overstretching.

2 **Rearview mirror** When you first get into a car, sit up straight and adjust the rearview mirror – this will act as a reminder every time you are tempted to slump behind the wheel.

3 **Seat height** If you experience aching in your accelerator leg when driving long distances, experiment with the height of the seat, as this may bring relief.

Shopping

When shopping, try to avoid being laden down with too many goods. Supermarket shopping, in particular, can be hazardous, because most of us buy trolley-loads of goods that either need to be carried, or lifted into a car

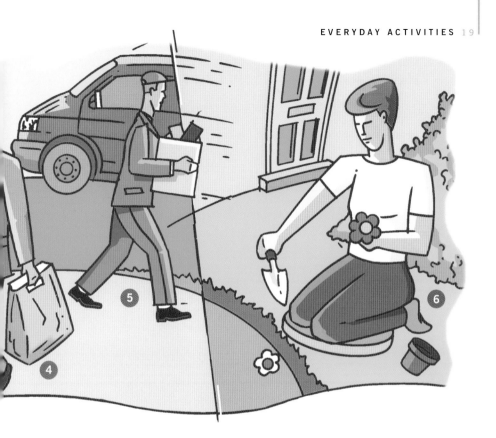

and lifted out at the other end. Trolleys themselves are often poorly designed and become increasingly difficult to push the more you add to them. Their depth also makes them difficult to unload at the checkout.

4 **Shopping quantities** Shop in smaller quantities if possible, or ask a friend to go with you to share the load. (See also lifting and carrying tips on pages 14–15.)

5 **Home-delivery service** If possible, arrange to have all the bulky items on your shopping list delivered by the store.

Gardening

Gardening can be back-breaking work, so try to vary the jobs and don't do too much at once. Keep your back straight and avoid bending as much as possible. Long-handled gardening implements can be useful. When digging, stand close to the area where you are working and try not to overload the fork or spade. Mowing can be heavy work, too, so choose a mower that is light and maneuverable. If you need to use a wheelbarrow, choose one that carries the load forward over the wheel.

6 **Planting and weeding** Kneeling to tend to your flowerbeds is a lot kinder to your back than bending.

THE **BACK-FRIENDLY HOME**

We spend a large proportion of our lives inside our homes, so it is important that we make them as back-friendly as possible. It is easy to take our surroundings for granted, however, and we may not even notice the potential danger zones. Poorly designed chairs, a soft, sagging mattress, wall cupboards that are too high, or work surfaces that are too low are all likely to lead to discomfort and back problems. Fortunately, there are many practical ways to make your home back-friendly.

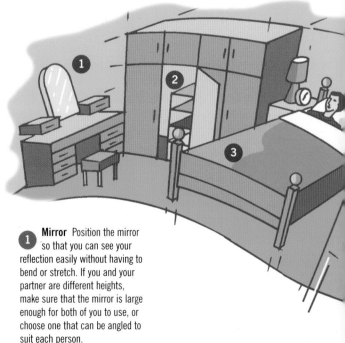

The bedroom

For a back-friendly bedroom, the most essential item is a good, firm mattress. It should provide enough support to maintain the healthy curves of the spine. Remember that having a very low bed, or a mattress on the floor, can be a struggle to get into and out of. Wardrobes, chests of drawers, and dressing tables need to be an appropriate height for easy access.

1 Mirror Position the mirror so that you can see your reflection easily without having to bend or stretch. If you and your partner are different heights, make sure that the mirror is large enough for both of you to use, or choose one that can be angled to suit each person.

2 **Wardrobe** Choose a wardrobe that is easy to open and close. The rail should be positioned so that you can reach your clothes comfortably. Avoid shelves that are too high, or use them to store items that you do not wear very often.

3 **Bed** A good mattress is vital. It should be firm, but allow absorption of the hips and shoulders. If your mattress is old and soft, try putting a board underneath it to give you more support. Avoid too many pillows.

The sitting room

Choose furniture that supports your back properly. Chairs and sofas should be comfortable, but still give adequate support to your lower back. Avoid oversoft or bucket-shaped chairs.

4 **Sofa and chairs** These should offer good support for your back and should not be too low, since this will make you slump. You should be able to sit with your hips against the back of the seat, with your feet flat on the floor.

5 **Television** Position the TV at eye level or higher, straight in front of you, so that you can see it without twisting your neck and body. You may have to angle some of the chairs to achieve this.

6 **Sound system** This should be easily accessible. Avoid having to bend or stretch unnecessarily to reach it.

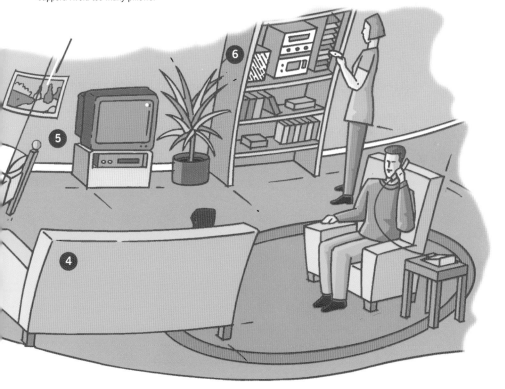

The bathroom

Plan your bathroom to avoid unnecessary bending or awkward twisting, and make sure that all surfaces are at the right height for their purpose. Maximize your bathroom's back-friendliness with a generous-sized bathtub that offers good support for your back, and a lavatory and basin of a suitable height. Make sure that towels and other items are easy to reach.

1 **Basin** The basin should be at an appropriate height with a mirror positioned above it, so that you can see your reflection without bending or stretching. If children are unable to reach, a sturdy box or low stool for them to stand on may help.

2 **Bathtub** You should be able to stretch out your legs in the bathtub. The bathtub should also have a sloping back, so that you can lie against it comfortably. Handles on the side are useful for getting in and out easily.

3 **Lavatory** Low-level lavatories may be difficult to sit down on or get up from. Wall-mounted flushes are easier to reach than chains that need pulling. Make sure that toilet tissue is kept within easy reaching distance.

The kitchen

Plan your kitchen so that the work surfaces and appliances are at the right height for their purpose and can be used comfortably. Keep everything that you use regularly within easy reach. You may find a tall stool useful, so that you can alternate between standing and sitting at the work surface.

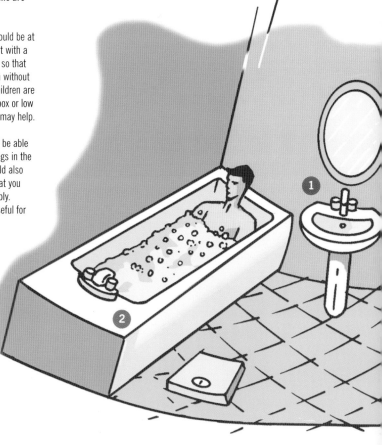

4 **Kitchen sink** You should be able to use the sink without stooping. If it is too low, raise the washing-up bowl to the required height by placing it on top of another, upturned bowl.

5 **Work surfaces** These should be at a comfortable height, so that your back is straight and your arms are at right angles to your body when you are working.

6 **Cupboards and shelves** Store items that you use regularly, particularly if heavy, in cupboards or on shelves that are within easy reach, to avoid undue bending or stretching.

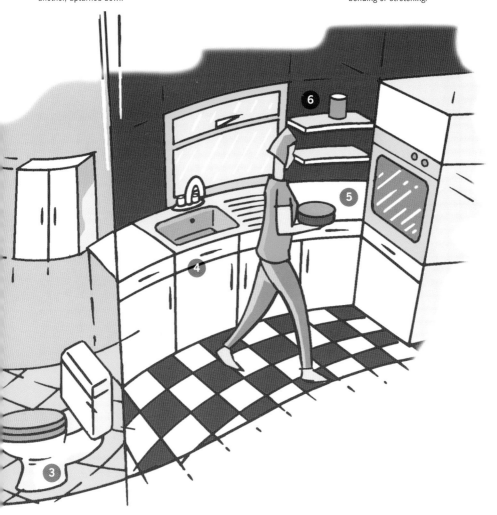

IN THE **WORKPLACE**

Workers in the United States and Europe take more time off for back problems than for any other health problem, with up to half the workforce being affected by back pain at some time in any given year, so it is worth thinking about the potential danger zones and what you can do to make life easier for your back. Sedentary workers, especially those who work at a computer screen for hours at a time, are particularly vulnerable to backache and back pain.

1 **Chair** Pull your chair right in under your desk, so that you do not have to crane forward.

2 **Legs and feet** Your lower legs should be at right angles to your thighs, with your feet flat on the floor. If not, use a footrest or a couple of telephone directories to support your feet. Do not store anything else under your desk; there should be nothing obstructing your leg movement.

3 **Breaks** Take regular breaks when using a computer screen; this will help to improve your concentration and prevent stiffness. Get up, stretch, and move around every half hour. See pages 54–57 for back stretches you can do in the office.

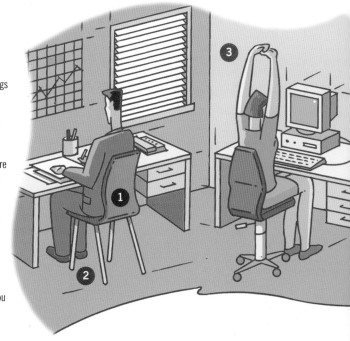

SITTING AT A COMPUTER: THE IDEAL POSITION

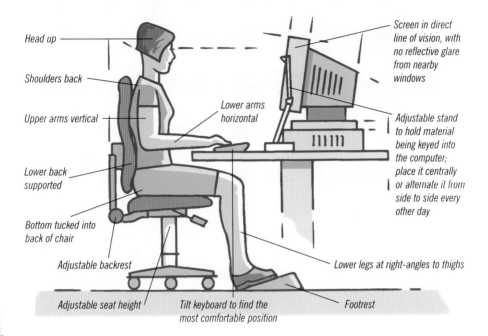

Head up

Shoulders back

Upper arms vertical

Lower arms horizontal

Lower back supported

Bottom tucked into back of chair

Adjustable backrest

Adjustable seat height

Tilt keyboard to find the most comfortable position

Footrest

Lower legs at right-angles to thighs

Screen in direct line of vision, with no reflective glare from nearby windows

Adjustable stand to hold material being keyed into the computer; place it centrally or alternate it from side to side every other day

ARE YOU AT RISK?

Common hazards in the workplace include:
- office chairs that are the wrong height for the desks, or that do not adequately support the lower back
- poor sitting posture
- computer screens or work areas that are badly positioned, forcing you to twist your neck uncomfortably
- constantly working in the same position or carrying out repetitive activities
- crooking the head to one side and tucking a telephone handset between the head and shoulder so that your hands are free to write or type

Other types of work

If your work is not office-based, there will be other factors to bear in mind. If your job entails standing for long periods of time, make sure that you are standing properly (see page 13) and shift your position regularly. If you lift things or drive as part of your work, make sure that you know how to do these activities in a back-friendly way (see pages 14–15 and 18).

PREGNANCY

During pregnancy, the back has to adapt to greater strain. The increasing size and weight of the baby can lead to a change in posture – many women lean back on the heels to compensate for the increased load at the front. The resulting hollow in the spine puts additional stress on the lower back and may force the upper back into a compromised position. The extra weight also causes the disks in the lower spine to compress more than usual, making the back more vulnerable to aches and pains.

1 **Poor posture** If you lean back on your heels, the resulting hollow in the small of your back will put extra stress on your spine. This becomes increasingly difficult to avoid as the pregnancy progresses and the baby grows larger and heavier.

2 **Good posture** Stand tall and relaxed, with your feet parallel and as wide apart as your hips. Imagine a thread running through your body from head to foot, drawing you upward. Always keep your shoulders relaxed and your knees loose rather than locked.

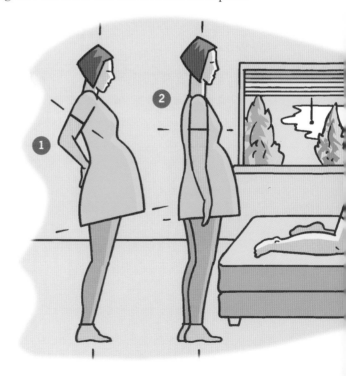

3 Getting up after lying down

In later pregnancy, if you sit up awkwardly after lying down, you can strain your back and stomach muscles. To get up, roll onto your side, draw your knees up, and use your arms to push yourself up sidewise. Swing your legs around, put your feet flat on the floor, then stand up slowly.

4 Getting up from a chair

Keeping your back straight, lean forward so that your body weight is balanced over your thighs. Place one foot slightly in front of the other and stand up slowly.

Rest and relaxation

To take the pressure off the spine during pregnancy, take frequent rests, lying on a bed or sofa. Placing a pillow between the knees can make lying on the side easier. Kneeling on all fours can also help to relieve pressure on the spine. For relaxation, massage can be very effective in relieving many of the stresses and discomforts of pregnancy (see pages 72–73).

Keep active

It is important to move around, as well as rest, during pregnancy in order to keep the spine flexible. Swimming is an excellent form of exercise for pregnant women, since it is gentle, promotes suppleness, and the body's weight is supported by the water. Other suitable activities include walking and dancing. Sensible exercising during pregnancy will help to avoid back strain, tone the body and prepare it for labor, and increase vitality.

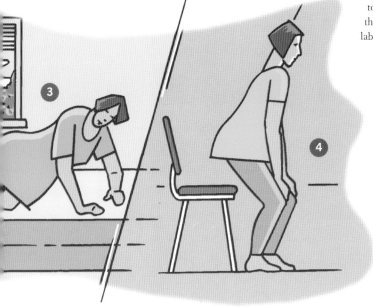

LIFESTYLE

A number of key lifestyle factors play an important role in helping to maintain a healthy back. These include weight and diet, fitness, stress, age, and travel. One of the most important things that you can do to ensure that your back stays strong is to maintain your ideal weight. An active lifestyle will also help to keep your back healthy and supple. Another common problem is stress – feeling stressed can have a detrimental effect on posture, causing stiffness and tension in the neck, shoulders, and back.

Weight and healthy eating

The more weight you carry around, the more pressure you are putting on the muscles and disks of your lower back. If you feel that you are overweight, try to change your eating patterns. A healthy diet includes plenty of fresh fruit, vegetables, whole grains, and some protein. Make sure that you have sufficient calcium in your diet – from milk, cheese, oily fish, and green leafy vegetables – to keep your bones healthy. In addition, since vertebral disks are 80 percent water, it is important to drink several glasses of water a day to keep them in working order.

A diet full of fresh fruits and vegetables will help to keep your bones strong and your weight at an ideal level for a healthy back.

Feeling fit

Try to build activity into your daily routine. Even simple changes, such as walking the children to school rather than driving them, or using the stairs at work rather than the elevator, can be effective ways of increasing your activity level.

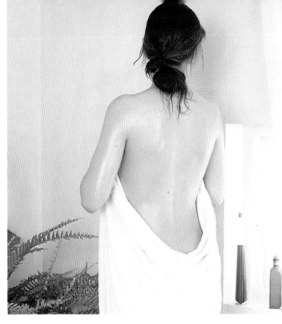

Stress can cause muscular tension and lead to poor posture. Always set aside a few minutes each day to relax and unwind.

De-stressing your life

Spend some time each day de-stressing yourself. A few minutes listening to music, stretching, meditating, or simply doing nothing at all can make all the difference between feeling focused and "in control" and feeling stressed (see chapter two for detailed guidance on relaxation techniques).

Getting older

By maintaining a healthy, active lifestyle, you can do a lot to prevent back problems in later life. However, it is important to bear in mind that what you can do comfortably without straining your back will gradually decrease as you get older, so it is vital that you learn and respect your new limits.

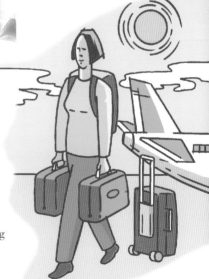

Travel tips

Make sure that your suitcases are not too heavy and distribute the weight evenly. Pack two small suitcases rather than one big one, and wherever possible, use luggage on wheels. Alternatively, pay a porter to help – it could work out a lot cheaper in the long run!

When traveling, carry two small suitcases rather than one large one. Better still, use luggage on wheels – it is a lot more back-friendly than carrying heavy cases.

EXERCISE AND **YOUR BACK**

Regular exercise not only improves the efficiency of the heart and lungs, and helps to prevent heart disease and other health problems, it also strengthens back muscles and improves the mobility of the spine. Walking, with a good rhythmical stride and your arms swinging loosely at your sides, helps to improve posture, and as you walk, your back muscles relax and contract. Swimming is another good form of exercise, both for your general health and for your spine, and is particularly beneficial if you suffer from back problems.

Swim to a healthy back

Swimming encourages mobility and strengthens back muscles. In addition, the water's buoyancy supports the body's weight, so you can exercise without putting strain on your spine. Front crawl and backstroke are the most effective strokes. Take care that you use the correct technique when swimming breaststroke.

1 Poor technique Try not to hold your head above water when swimming breaststroke, because this puts pressure on the neck and the top part of the back.

2 Good technique Keep your head below water and your spine straight while breathing out. You may find that wearing a pair of goggles helps.

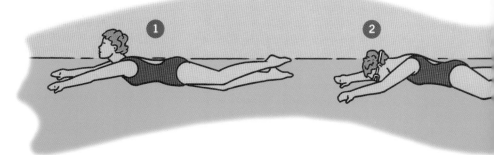

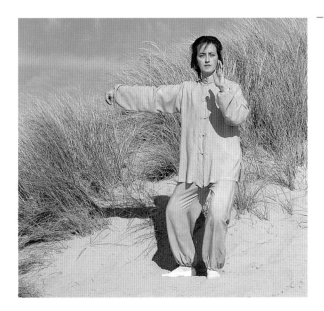

3 **Taking a breath** Bring your head and upper body above water for gulps of air every alternate stroke. Try to keep your back as straight as possible.

Tai chi and yoga are good forms of gentle exercise that can actively benefit your back and improve your general sense of well-being.

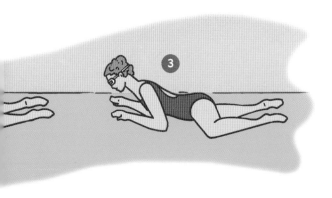

TAKE CARE

Most sports and games are good for you, but you may need to be cautious with some.

- Jogging and running can be bad for your back if you run on a hard surface, because shockwaves from the impact can jar the spine and even compress the disks; wearing well-cushioned shoes or jogging on a softer surface, such as grass, will help to absorb the impact
- The vigorous twisting actions in golf, and serving in racket games such as squash and tennis, can strain your back if you overdo them, or have a poor technique; try to improve your technique — gradually! — and be aware that racket sports also tend to build up strength on one side of the body only
- Cycling is a great form of exercise, but cycling for long periods of time on a bike with drop-handle bars can put stress on the back; ride an upright bike if possible
- Activities where your body might be subjected to a lot of force, such as contact sports and trampolining, are not advisable if you have back problems

HOW TO **EXERCISE**

Exercising your back can relieve both acute (short-term) and chronic (long-term) back pain, and help to prevent it from recurring. Exercising does not have to mean taking part in a formal class or playing a team sport – you can exercise very effectively in your own home. On pages 34–57 you will find a home exercise routine that will help to keep your back mobile and strong, plus some stretches that you can do in your workplace.

When to exercise

Even after an attack of acute back pain, start to do some gentle exercise as soon as you are able. The sooner you start, the quicker your recovery. If you are in any doubt, seek professional advice and always stop if what you are doing hurts. There may be a little stiffness the next day if you are out of condition, but this should not stop you from exercising. A hot bath will help to ease any stiffness.

Footwear

If you are doing any type of exercise that involves your feet repeatedly hitting a hard surface, such as jogging, make sure your shoes have a well-cushioned sole and a thick heel to lessen the impact on your legs and spine. For gentler exercise, such as yoga, bare feet are best.

Clothing

Choose loose-fitting clothing, such as a track suit, baggy shorts, leggings, sweatshirt, and T-shirt, that is not restrictive and moves when you move. Look for items made from natural fibers that allow your skin to breathe rather than synthetic materials.

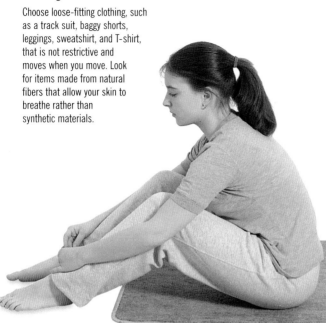

Where to exercise

Choose a quiet place where you will not be disturbed and where there is enough room to move freely. Play some soothing music; this will help you to keep your movements smooth, slow, and steady. The music will also help you to relax and may make exercising more enjoyable.

How much to exercise

If you are not used to exercising, start slowly and build up a regular routine gradually. Do not exercise too much too soon. Suddenly taking up a vigorous but erratic program of exercise can lead to injury, so try to exercise at roughly the same time every day. It will soon become a habit and you will reap the benefits more quickly.

DOS AND DON'TS

It is important to follow a few simple rules when taking up any form of exercise.

- Start slowly and build up gradually
- Choose a form of exercise that you enjoy – you will be much more likely to keep it up
- Always warm up beforehand and cool down afterwards with 5–10 minutes of gentle stretching exercises; you will not feel so stiff the next day and your spine will benefit from the stretching
- Slip on a pair of trousers and a sweatshirt once you have stopped exercising, to avoid your body cooling down too quickly and your muscles becoming stiff
- If any activity or exercise makes your back hurt, stop and do some strengthening exercises instead (see the exercise routine on pages 34–57)

STRETCH FOR A **HEALTHY BACK**

This program of gentle stretching exercises will help to strengthen the muscles, joints, and ligaments in your back. Your back will become more flexible, the chance of back strain or injury will be reduced, and your breathing and circulation will be improved. You will also feel far more relaxed – and don't be surprised to find that you have lots more energy, and feel and look better than ever before. Spend 10–20 minutes stretching every day if possible; if not, try to do the exercises at least three times a week.

How to follow the program

The program consists of specific exercises for each part of the back. Here are a few simple guidelines to help you gain maximum benefit from the program.
• Follow all of the exercises on pages 35–47 in sequence if time allows (it should take about 20 minutes)
• Alternatively, select one or two from each section for a quick 10-minute workout
• Try the advanced poses on pages 48–49 only when you have mastered the basic exercises
• If you have just a few spare minutes and feel in need of a stretch, choose the quick-and-easy exercises on pages 50–53
• Finally, the stretches on pages 54–57 have been especially devised for in the workplace

Flexibility

It does not matter if you are not very flexible to begin with. Start by holding the poses for a short time, then gradually build up your stamina and hold the poses for longer. You may find that some of the exercises are easier on one side of your body. Don't let it stop you from doing exercises on the difficult side. Breathe and be patient. Don't give up if you feel a little stiff at first. You will soon reap the benefits.

WARNING
If you experience acute pain, or have any doubts about the health of your back, consult a medical practitioner before embarking on any course of exercise.

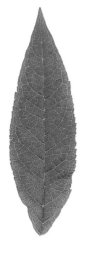

WARMING UP AND **COOLING DOWN**

Whatever form of exercise you take, or whatever part of your body you are exercising, it is important to start by doing some gentle stretching to warm up your muscles, and to finish in the same way to prevent any stiffness the next day. These poses can also be used to give your body a rest at any stage in the exercise program, or whenever you want to relax.

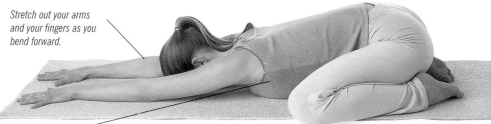

Stretch out your arms and your fingers as you bend forward.

Rest your forehead and upper chest on the floor if you can.

Embryo

Sit with your bottom on your heels and your knees spread apart. Breathe in, and slowly bend your torso forward between your knees. Breathe out. Relax and breathe normally. Hold the pose for a couple of minutes, then slowly return to an upright position.

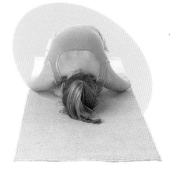

Alternative embryo

Start with your knees together rather than spread apart. As you lean forward, slowly bring your arms back toward your toes. Keep your arms relaxed and palms facing upward.

DO
• use this as a resting pose at any point between exercises

DON'T
• get up too quickly

GOOD FOR
• stretching the spine
• resting in flexion after extension exercises

Cool cat

Begin on your hands and knees, with your weight evenly distributed. Slowly draw your back up into an arch, with your head down, and breathe in. Hold the position for five seconds, then breathe out. Slowly allow the small of your back to sink into a U-shape, pulling your head up to look toward the ceiling at the same time. Hold for five seconds. Repeat both steps 10 times.

▼ 1 Starting on all fours, pull your back up into an arch and drop your head forward. Hold for five seconds.

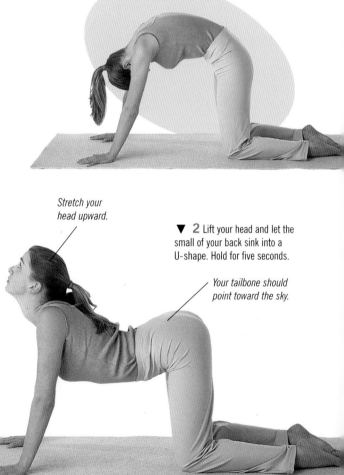

Stretch your head upward.

▼ 2 Lift your head and let the small of your back sink into a U-shape. Hold for five seconds.

Your tailbone should point toward the sky.

DO
- remember to breathe
- hold each part of the pose for a full five seconds

DON'T
- overstretch – take the pose to a comfortable limit

GOOD FOR
- flexion and extension warm-ups
- improving the flexibility of the small muscles and ligaments of the spine

Dog pose

Crouch on all fours, then push your bottom upward by straightening your legs and arms. Without bending your knees, drop your head toward the floor and press your heels downward. Breathe in. As you breathe out, push your tailbone toward the sky. Spread your fingers and rotate the outside of your elbows toward the front. Lift your body weight at the shoulders and hold for 30 seconds, breathing normally.

DO
• relax your head and neck

DON'T
• forget to breathe

GOOD FOR
• stretching the large muscles of the back, particularly across the neck and shoulders
• stretching the hamstrings on the back of the thighs and opening up the pelvic area

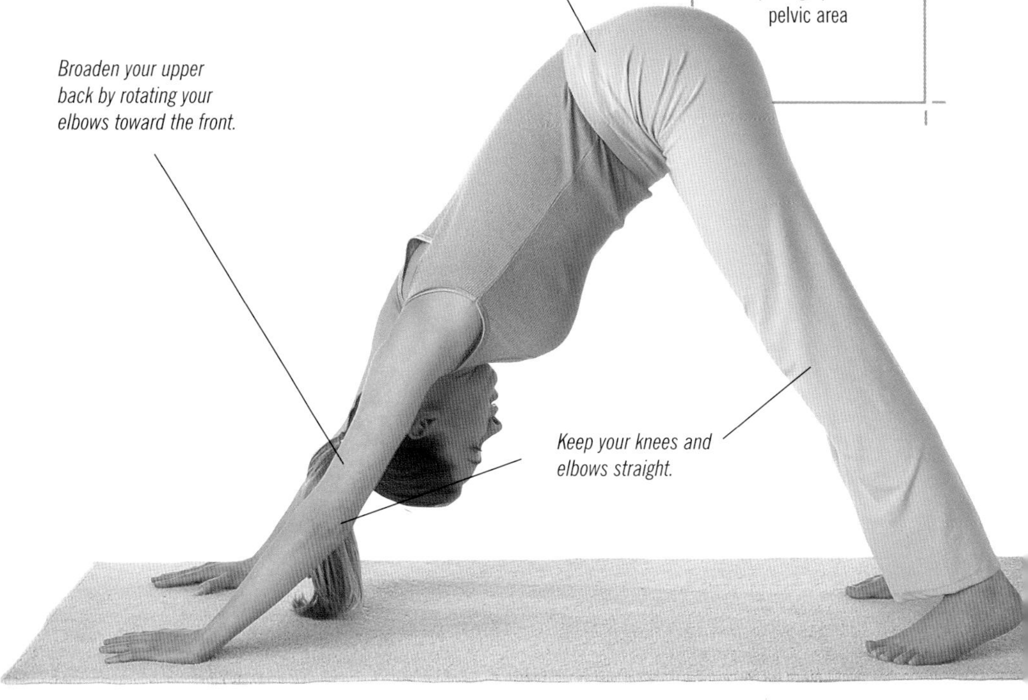

Lift your body weight at your shoulders and tailbone.

Broaden your upper back by rotating your elbows toward the front.

Keep your knees and elbows straight.

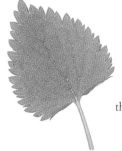

LOWER **BACK**

The lower back is a common site for back pain, because many of the deeper muscles of the back originate in the small area around the back of the pelvis. These exercises will help to relax these muscles, prevent compression of the lower back, and stretch the whole spine.

Cobra

Lie face down on the floor with your arms bent and your palms alongside your chest. Breathe in, and looking up, press down on your palms and stretch your torso upward. Breathe out, rotate the inside of your elbows toward the front, raise your breastbone, and draw back your head. Gently tighten your buttocks and hold the position for 20 seconds, breathing normally. Breathe out, relax your arms, and allow your torso to sink slowly to the floor.

DO
• tighten your buttocks to prevent compression in the lower back

DON'T
• constrict your neck or strain your throat
• hold your breath

GOOD FOR
• overall stretching
• strengthening chest muscles, and firming breasts and neck
• releasing abdominal tension

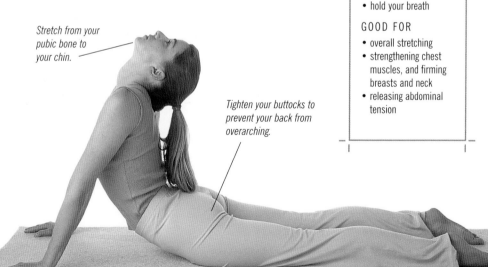

Stretch from your pubic bone to your chin.

Tighten your buttocks to prevent your back from overarching.

Kickbacks

Starting on your hands and knees, arch your back up toward the ceiling, bring your left leg in toward your body, and drop your head toward your bent knee. Then lift your head up so that you are facing straight ahead and gently extend your left leg backward. Keep the extended leg slightly bent at the knee. Repeat 10 times, then do the same with your right leg.

▲ 1 Starting on all fours, arch your back, bring one leg in toward your chest, and drop your head toward your knee.

DO
• maintain rhythm

DON'T
• be overzealous and never overstretch

GOOD FOR
• toning the whole back, neck, and hips

▼ 2 Lift your head up and extend your leg backward.

Remember to lift your head as you extend your leg.

Keep your extended leg slightly bent to increase the stretch on your lower back.

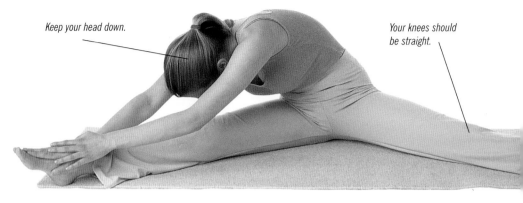

Keep your head down.

Your knees should be straight.

Sitting splits

Sit with your legs as far apart as is comfortable. Breathe in and stretch both your arms above your head. Breathe out and slowly stretch down toward your right foot with both arms. Hold for five seconds, breathing out. Gently return to the sitting position. Stretch up again and repeat the exercise on the opposite side.

Advanced sitting splits

Try these advanced sitting splits once you have mastered the basic technique. They are good for stretching the ribcage and its muscles. Sitting with your legs apart, bend to the side and place your right elbow on the floor in front of you. Breathe in, and bring your left arm over your head toward your right foot until you can feel the stretch along the left side of your body. Hold for five seconds, breathing out. Repeat on the opposite side.

DO
- hold your calf if you cannot reach your foot, or use a belt around the arch of your foot to help pull yourself down
- relax your head and neck

DON'T
- let your knees bend
- move quickly

GOOD FOR
- stretching buttocks
- decongesting the pelvic area and regulating menstrual flow

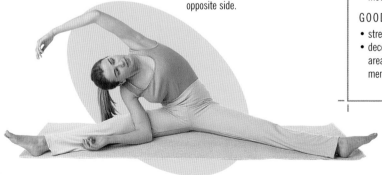

Lumbar roll

Lie on your back with legs outstretched and arms bent, both elbows on the floor, palms facing upward. Lift one leg, bending it at the knee. Slowly move the bent leg across your body, down toward the opposite side. Breathing normally, hold the pose for 30 seconds. Slowly raise your leg and return it to its original position. Repeat the pose on the other side.

DO
• move your legs slowly

DON'T
• force it – remember, it's the journey, not the destination that counts!

GOOD FOR
• releasing the sacroiliac joints and lumbar spine
• slimming the waistline

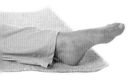

As you relax, let your knee fall closer to the floor.

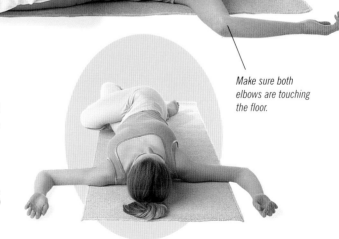

Make sure both elbows are touching the floor.

Advanced lumbar roll

Once you have mastered the basic lumbar roll, try this more advanced version. Place your arms as before, but wrap your outstretched legs around each other. Gently roll the tangle of legs to one side. Breathe in and stretch both elbows to the floor. Hold the pose for 15 seconds, breathing normally. Slowly return to a central position, then repeat on the opposite side.

Sit-ups

Sit-ups help to strengthen the stomach muscles, which in turn improves posture and increases the strength and flexibility of the lower back. It is essential that sit-ups be performed correctly, because injury can result if they are done poorly. First, do five straight sit-ups, then five diagonal sit-ups. Gradually build up to 10 sit-ups of each kind. Once you have mastered both these techniques, try the advanced sit-ups.

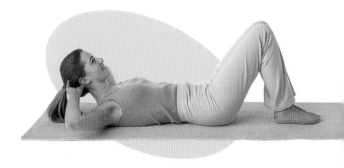

Straight sit-ups

▲ **1** Lie with your knees bent and feet apart. Put your hands behind your head, with your fingers spread and thumbs pointing down.

▼ **2** Breathe in and slowly lift your head and shoulders toward your knees to the count of four. Breathe out and lie back down to a count of four. Repeat four times.

Lift your head and shoulders off the floor.

Feel the abdominal muscles contract and shorten, pulling you up.

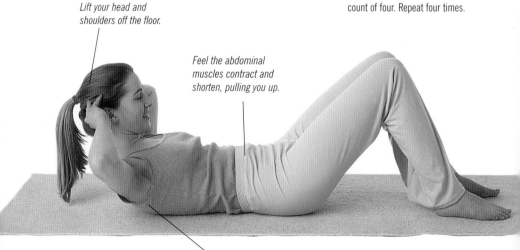

Don't lift your body too far.

Diagonal sit-ups

Lift your feet into the air with your knees bent. With your hands behind your head, breathe in and lift one elbow toward the opposite knee. Breathe out and release. Come straight back up with the other elbow, toward the opposite knee. Repeat four times on each side.

Keep your knees bent and feet off the floor.

Spread your fingers out on the back of your head.

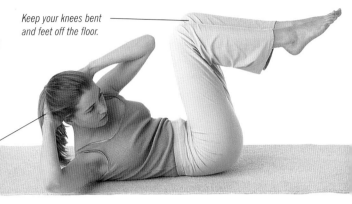

DO
- keep space for an imaginary orange under your chin as you pull up
- build up the number of sit-ups to 10 repeats of each exercise as you get stronger

DON'T
- perform the basic sit-ups with straight legs – this can strain the lower back
- contract your buttock muscles

GOOD FOR
- toning and strengthening stomach muscles
- slimming the waistline
- stretching the lower back muscles

Keep your head level and look straight ahead.

Keep your legs straight.

Don't curve your back.

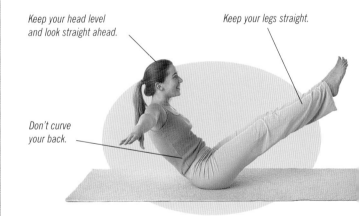

Advanced sit-ups

Do not try this advanced technique until you have mastered the basic straight and diagonal sit-ups. Lie on your back with your arms by your sides. Breathe in and lift your legs and arms up so that your body forms a V-shape, then move your arms out to the sides. Hold this position for two seconds, then gently lower your body back to the floor. Rest for four seconds, then repeat. Aim to build up to 10 repeats.

MID-**BACK**

Pain in the mid-back area is often caused by poor posture – for example, if the back is too straight, or curved over into a stooped position, this can be a result of poor posture. The following exercises can help to remedy postural problems and strengthen and stretch the mid-back area.

Turn your head away from your outstretched arm.

Twist

Sit cross-legged on the floor. Take your right foot and put it over your left knee, which should rest on the floor. Put your left arm over the raised right knee, and using this as a lever, turn toward your right-hand side. Use your right arm for balance. Breathe in. As you breathe out, try to turn even farther toward the right. Breathe in and return to a central position. Repeat the exercise on the other side, then repeat once more on each side.

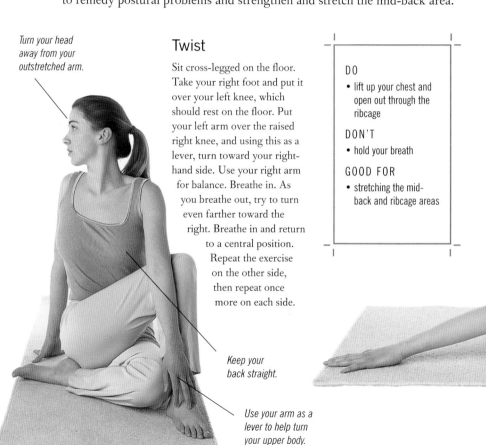

Keep your back straight.

Use your arm as a lever to help turn your upper body.

DO
- lift up your chest and open out through the ribcage

DON'T
- hold your breath

GOOD FOR
- stretching the mid-back and ribcage areas

Ribcage stretch

Kneel on the floor and bend forward so that your head touches the floor. Stretch out your left arm above your head and thread your right arm underneath and across your body. Raise your bottom, and turn your head and shoulders to face your right arm. Hold this position for 30 seconds, then repeat on the other side.

DO
- feel the stretch through the mid-back area
- enjoy this exercise as a resting pose

DON'T
- twist your upper body too far around

GOOD FOR
- opening up the ribcage area
- easing shoulder blade stiffness

Your tailbone should point to the sky.

Aim to create a good diagonal line with your upper body.

Face the same way as your outstretched arm.

Rest your arm loosely on the floor.

UPPER **BACK AND NECK**

The upper back and neck are prone to stiffness and tension, particularly
if posture is poor. These exercises will help to release tension and
keep your upper back, neck, and shoulders strong and supple, as
well as stretch your whole spine.

Deep dorsal stretch

Kneel on the floor in front of
a chair. Interlock your
forearms and bend forward so
that they rest on the edge of
the chair seat. Drop your head
forward. Exhale and allow
your chest to sink toward the
floor. Hold for 15 seconds.

DO
• keep breathing steadily

DON'T
• come up too quickly

GOOD FOR
• shoulder and neck
  stiffness
• easing tension in the
  shoulder blades

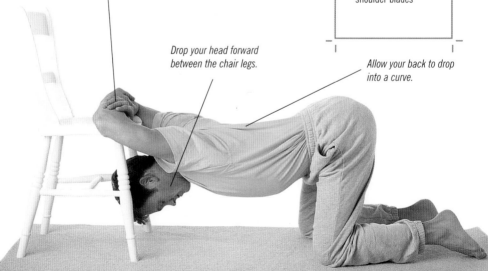

*Rest your forearms
on the edge of the
chair seat.*

*Drop your head forward
between the chair legs.*

*Allow your back to drop
into a curve.*

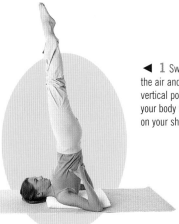

◀ 1 Swing your legs into the air and hold them in a vertical position. Most of your body weight should be on your shoulders.

DO
• go into the position slowly and gently

DON'T
• attempt to bring your legs over your head until you are confident with the shoulder stand
• constrict the throat and chest – press down with your arms and lift the chest up

GOOD FOR
• releasing shoulder tension
• improving body balance and awareness

Navel gazer

Place a folded towel on the floor. Lie with your shoulders and upper back on the towel and your head over the edge. Lift up your legs and torso into a shoulder stand. Bend the elbows and use your hands to support your lower back. Breathe normally. Breathing out, lower your legs to the floor beyond your head. Bend your knees and bring them close to your ears. Keep breathing rhythmically. Hold this position for 30 seconds.

▼ 2 Keeping your legs straight, bring them down to the floor beyond your head.

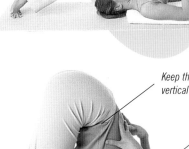

▶ 3 Bend your knees so that one knee rests beside each ear.

Keep the torso as vertical as possible.

Continue to use your arms to support your lower back.

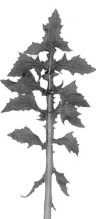

ADVANCED **EXERCISES**

If you have worked your way through the basic exercise program and are ready for a new challenge, try these slightly more advanced poses. They are designed for those who have already built up their spinal flexibility. Do not attempt these exercises without first becoming adept at the basic program.

Arabesque

Stand tall with your legs together. Stretch your right arm out in front of you at shoulder level. Put your weight onto your right leg and bend the knee slightly. Slowly raise your left leg behind you and grasp the ankle with your left hand. Bend forward, using your outstretched arms to maintain your balance. Hold the pose for up to 30 seconds. Repeat the exercise, stretching your left arm out in front of you and raising your right leg behind you.

Keep your outstretched arm as straight as possible.

Balance the weight of your torso between your two arms.

Grasp your ankle with your hand, keeping your other leg vertical.

DO
• warm up first

DON'T
• be discouraged if you lose your balance — keep trying!

GOOD FOR
• stretching the whole spine
• balance and poise

Bridge

Lie on your back with your legs a few inches apart and your arms by your sides. Bring your knees up. Elongate your neck. Breathing out, push your pelvis up toward the ceiling. Breathe in, lifting up through the chest. Bend your arms and place your hands under your hips for support. Hold the pose, breathing normally, for one minute. Release your arms, breathe out, and gently lower your torso to the floor.

DO
- warm up well first
- work your thigh muscles

DON'T
- compress through the throat area; instead, lift up through the chest

GOOD FOR
- stretching the lumbar spine
- correcting rounded shoulders
- releasing tension in the neck and shoulders

▼ **1** Lie on the floor with arms by your sides, feet apart, and knees drawn up.

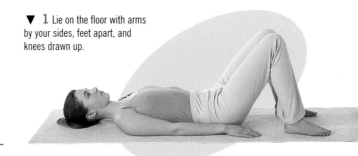

Use your hands to support your lower back.

▶ **2** Lift your pelvis up and support your hips with your hands.

Push your pelvis upward to form a bridge.

Keep your feet flat on the floor.

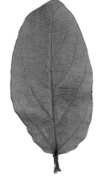

QUICK-AND-EASY **STRETCHES**

These exercises, as the name suggests, are designed for those occasions when you do not have much time, but feel that your back would benefit from a quick, simple exercise or two.

Rock'n'roll

Lie on your back. Bend your knees up toward your chest and wrap your arms around them. Lift your head, forming your body into a ball. Rock yourself backward and forward, keeping your head tucked in and your knees in toward your chest.

Wrap your arms around your knees to bring them up to your chest.

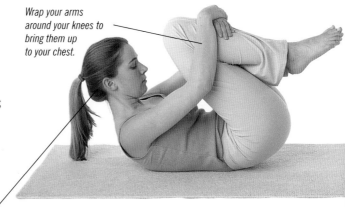

Lift your head to meet your knees so that you are curled up in a ball.

▲ **1** Wrap your arms around your legs so that your body curls into a ball shape.

▶ **2** Swing backward and forward, massaging your whole spine against the floor.

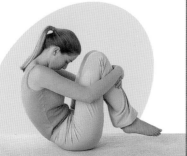

DO
• put some padding onto the floor, such as a folded blanket, especially if you are thin

DON'T
• get up too quickly afterwards

GOOD FOR
• an overall spinal massage

Standing twists

Stand with your feet apart and legs straight. Raise your arms in front of you and cross your forearms at shoulder level. Twist your torso around, looking back over one shoulder. Only twist as far as is comfortable and don't jerk your body – try to keep the movement smooth. Return to the front position. Do five twists on each side.

▼ **1** With your forearms crossed at shoulder height, swing around in one direction.

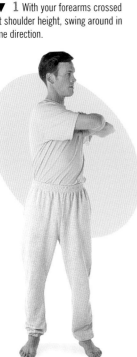

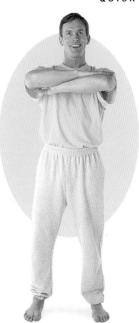

▲ **2** Come back to the front position, then do four more twists in the same direction.

Twist your head and arms around to look back over your shoulder.

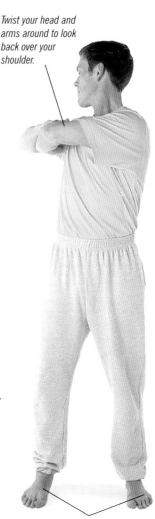

Keep your feet shoulder-width apart.

▲ **3** Swing in the opposite direction in the same way a total of five times.

DO
- keep your back and legs straight

DON'T
- be too vigorous – this exercise is designed to be a quick stretch

GOOD FOR
- stretching the upper back and ribcage

The bends

These simple flexion and extension exercises are ideal for stretching the whole spine and can be performed almost anywhere. Start by performing five back bends, then 10 front bends, and finish with five side bends on each side. Take care not to bend too far – only stretch as far as is comfortable, increasing the stretch only after your spine has become more flexible.

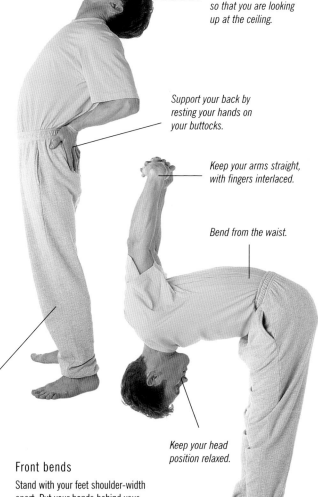

Bend backward slightly, so that you are looking up at the ceiling.

Support your back by resting your hands on your buttocks.

Keep your arms straight, with fingers interlaced.

Bend from the waist.

Keep your head position relaxed.

Back bends

Stand with your feet shoulder-width apart. Rest your hands on your buttocks, breathing in. As you breathe out, look up and bend back a little. Breathe in and come up. Repeat four more times.

Keep your legs straight and your feet apart.

Front bends

Stand with your feet shoulder-width apart. Put your hands behind your back and interlace your fingers, breathing in. Breathe out and bend forward, lifting your arms up over your head. Breathe in and come up. Repeat nine more times.

Side bends

Stand with your feet around one-and-a-half shoulder-widths apart and breathe in. Breathing out, run your right hand down the side of your right thigh. To increase the stretch, raise your left arm over your head. Come up and repeat four more times on the same side. Repeat on the other side.

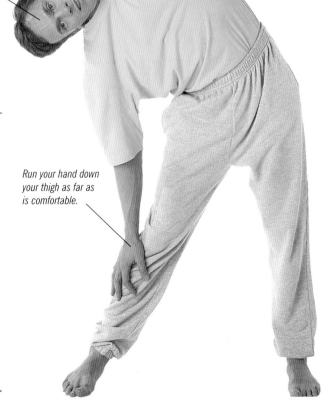

Lift your arm above your head.

Turn your head to the side, as if to look at the underside of your arm, if you wish to increase the stretch.

Run your hand down your thigh as far as is comfortable.

DO
- the exercise often   a good, quick stretch on a regular basis makes all the difference
- remember to stretch both sides of the body

DON'T
- overstretch – the poses should stretch you, but remain comfortable
- overbalance

GOOD FOR
- an overall stretch of the back

EXERCISES FOR THE **OFFICE**

These exercises can all be carried out in a seated position, so they are particularly suitable for performing in an office – in fact, on any occasion when you are sitting for any length of time and feel the need to stretch your back.

Keep your arms straight as you stretch upward.

Look straight ahead.

Upward stretch

Sitting down, interlace your fingers in front of you. Lift your arms up above your head, keeping the elbows straight and turning your palms to face the ceiling. Hold the position for 30 seconds, breathing normally. Bring your arms down slowly.

Keep your feet firmly on the ground.

DO
- remember to stretch your torso upward

DON'T
- look up – keep facing forward

GOOD FOR
- relaxation
- an overall stretch

Seated bends

You can perform bends from a sitting position quite easily. They are particularly effective for releasing tension in the upper back area. Start each exercise sitting on a chair, looking straight ahead with your feet flat on the floor.

Rest your hands on the floor.

Forward bends

Breathe out and bend forward, so that your hands are resting palms upward on the floor. Put your head between your knees. Hold for one minute or longer if you have time.

Keep your bottom flat on the chair.

Bend right over so that your head is near the floor.

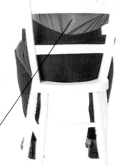

Keep your forearms crossed above your head as you bend.

Side bends

Lift your arms above your head and cross your forearms. Breathing out, gently bend to one side, stretching as you go. Breathe in and come up. Repeat on the other side. Repeat four more times on each side.

Bend from the waist.

DO

- keep breathing
- stay relaxed
- keep your feet flat on the ground and several inches apart

DON'T

- force your back to stretch farther than is comfortable
- overbalance

GOOD FOR

- an overall stretch
- releasing tension in the upper back
- any occasion when you are sitting for long periods of time

Arm wrap

Sit with both arms raised in front of you, upper arms at shoulder level and elbows bent so that your forearms are in front of your face. Interlace your forearms by putting your left elbow over your right one and linking hands. Keep your elbows bent at right angles and at shoulder height. Hold for 30 seconds, then interlace your arms in the opposite way.

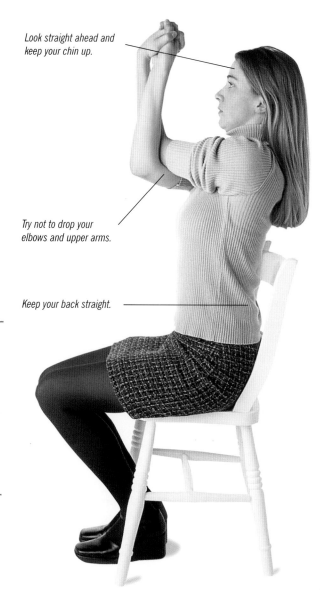

Look straight ahead and keep your chin up.

Try not to drop your elbows and upper arms.

Keep your back straight.

DO
- practice this exercise – it will get easier to do

DON'T
- hunch your shoulders

GOOD FOR
- stretching the upper back

Sitting twist

Sit sidewise in your chair with your left hip against the back of the chair. Breathe out and turn to the left, holding the back of the chair with both hands. Turn as far as you can, pushing with your left hand and pulling with your right. Turn your head to the side and look over your left shoulder. Relax, then repeat on the right-hand side.

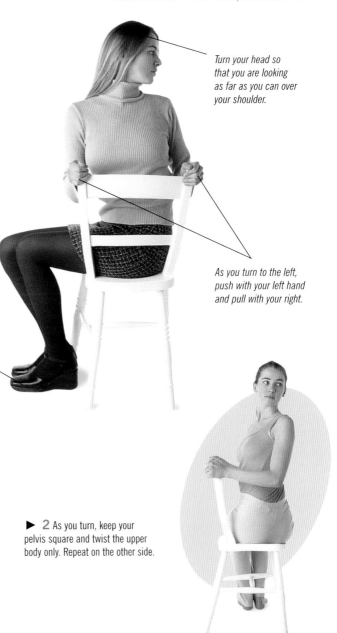

Turn your head so that you are looking as far as you can over your shoulder.

▶ **1** Sitting in a sidewise position, grasp the back of the chair and twist your upper body around.

As you turn to the left, push with your left hand and pull with your right.

Keep your legs and feet together.

DO
- lift up through the chest

DON'T
- allow the waist to compress

GOOD FOR
- releasing a tight mid- and upper back
- easing stiffness in the shoulder blades

▶ **2** As you turn, keep your pelvis square and twist the upper body only. Repeat on the other side.

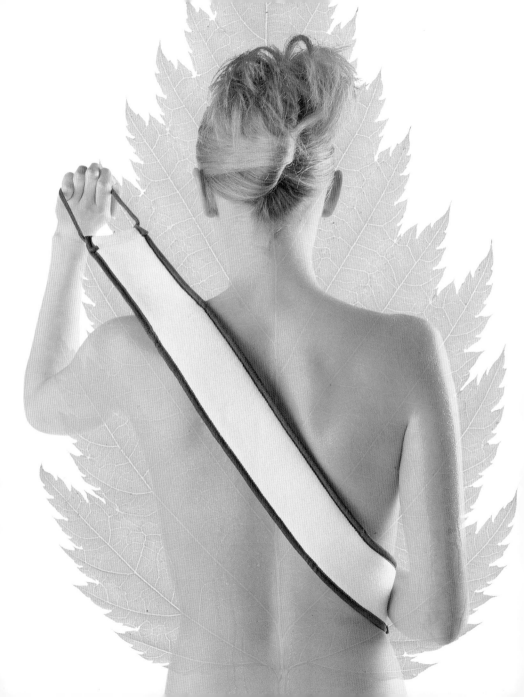

Relaxation and Beauty Treatments

RELAXATION

IS AN ESSENTIAL PART

OF BACK CARE. THIS CHAPTER

FOCUSES ON MASSAGE AND OTHER

RELAXATION TECHNIQUES, ALL OF

WHICH CAN HELP TO RELIEVE TENSION

AND IMPROVE OUR SENSE OF WELL-

BEING. THERE ARE ALSO BEAUTY

TREATMENTS TO HELP KEEP

YOUR BACK IN TIP-TOP

CONDITION.

THE **ART OF RELAXATION**

By cultivating a calm and peaceful state of mind, you will be able to handle the stresses and strains of everyday life much more easily. Two of the most popular and effective relaxation techniques are yoga and visualization. In the yoga life pose, you learn to observe the body's processes and let go of tension; the visualization technique helps you to transport yourself to a stress-free time or place, which promotes a strong sense of well-being.

Visualization

Sit on an upright chair or on the floor. Close your eyes and allow your head to balance comfortably between your shoulders. Wriggle your shoulders to release any tension, then bring your hands together on your lap. Listen to the gentle rhythm of your breathing. As you breathe out, repeat to yourself: *"I am at peace."* When you are truly at ease, imagine a time or place when everything felt good and in harmony. A summer vacation, perhaps, with the warmth of the sun on your body and the sound of the ocean lapping in the distance. Step inside the scene and feel yourself as part of it. Let it flow all around you. Stay in your visualization for as long as you wish, until you choose to return.

Yoga: The life pose

▶ 1 Sit on the floor with your knees bent. Lean backward and rest your body weight on your elbows with your palms face down.

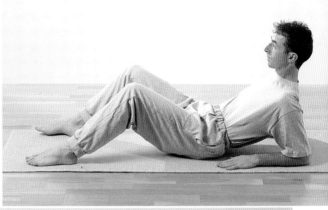

▼ 2 Slowly lower your back until it is as flat as possible against the floor. Straighten your arms and legs, and move your feet well apart.

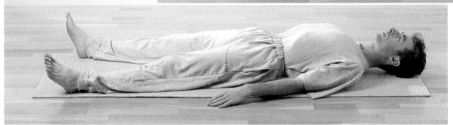

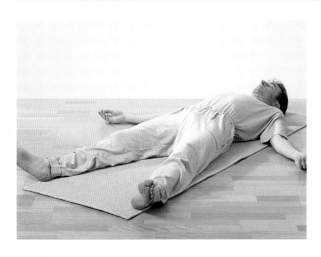

◀ 3 Move your arms away from your body, rolling your palms upward. Close your eyes and concentrate on your breathing pattern. Observe how the stomach rises as you breathe in and falls as you breathe out. Feel your muscles relax. Think about the various parts of your body, looking for areas of tension. At first, your mind is likely to wander, but this technique will become easier with practice. Hold the pose for five minutes, gradually building up to 15–20 minutes.

AROMATHERAPY

Aromatherapy uses aromatic and therapeutic essential oils to help you unwind and relax. The oils are extracted from plants – often well-known medicinal herbs – using a process known as distillation. Aromatherapy works in two ways: the oils themselves are absorbed through the skin into the circulatory system, and the oils' scents are transmitted directly to the brain via the olfactory nerves when inhaled. One of the simplest and most pleasurable ways of using essential oils is to add a few drops to your bath water, but you can use them in a variety of other ways.

Diluting essential oils

With the exception of lavender oil and tea tree oil, essential oils should not be applied directly to the skin. Dilute about 20 drops of essential oil in 2fl oz (50ml) of base oil, such as peach, almond, grapeseed, sunflower, safflower, or coconut oil. Store the diluted oil in an airtight dark glass bottle and keep it out of the sun in a cool, dry place. The refrigerator is ideal.

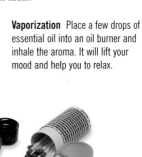

Vaporization Place a few drops of essential oil into an oil burner and inhale the aroma. It will lift your mood and help you to relax.

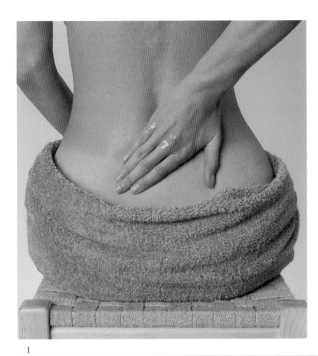

Massage Having an aromatherapy massage is the ideal way to release tight muscles, relax the body, and calm the mind (see pages 64–75 for massage techniques).

COMPRESSES

These contain essential oils to help ease aching muscles. Put a little oil into some hot water; it will form a film on the surface of the water. Place a cloth over the film, then lift it out and apply it to your back. (See also page 81.)

OILS FOR ACHES AND PAINS

Essential oils that are good for dealing with aches and pains include:
- birch
- lemongrass
- camomile
- marjoram
- rosemary
- juniper
- lavender

WARNING

If you are pregnant, or have epilepsy or high blood pressure, check with a qualified aromatherapist before using essential oils.

OILS TO RELIEVE STRESS

Essential oils that are good for relieving stress, which is often a factor in back pain, include:
- bergamot
- jasmine
- lavender
- lemongrass
- neroli
- patchouli
- ylang ylang

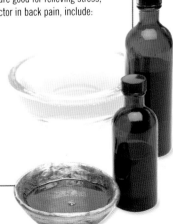

MASSAGE

Massage is an ancient healing art. Archeological discoveries indicate that prehistoric people massaged ointments and herbs into their bodies for healing purposes. Today, the increasingly fast pace at which we live has encouraged many people to rediscover the benefits of massage. Massage promotes relaxation and well-being; invigorates the body and mind; releases tension in muscles and joints; relieves pain; improves circulation; helps with the drainage of excess fluid and toxins from the body; and is the ideal way to introduce essential oils into the skin.

Effleurage

The basic stroke used in the massage routines on the following pages is effleurage, a long, slow, rhythmic movement, often described as stroking. Place the flat of your hands on the area to be massaged, fingers together and fingertips turned slightly upward, and rhythmically stroke the skin. Always effleurage toward the heart and increase the pressure as you stroke. Although effleurage is most commonly performed with the flat of the hand, it can also be done with the heel of the hand, the thumb, and the fist.

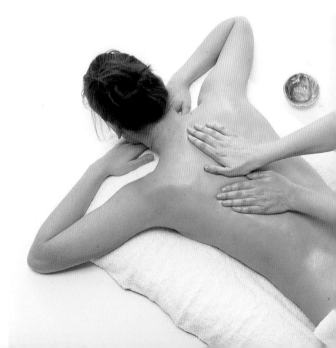

Preparation

Professional masseurs use a special bench for clients to lie on, but good alternatives include a foam rubber mat, a futon, or even the floor (beds are usually not firm enough). Cover the area with a large cotton sheet and spread a large towel over the top. Have extra towels and a pillow to hand. When being massaged, it is best to be completely naked. The parts of the body not being worked on should be covered with towels. The room needs to be warmer than usual and the lighting subdued. Shut the windows if there is traffic noise and close the drapes. Choose a time when you will not be disturbed, and unplug the phone or switch on the answerphone. Either work silently or play some soothing background music.

Getting started

Always use a massage oil so that the hands flow smoothly over the skin. Choose a vegetable oil, such as grapeseed, sunflower, or safflower oil, or sweet almond oil. For an aromatherapy massage, add a few drops of essential oil to the base oil (see pages 62–63). If you are giving the massage, make sure that you are familiar with any step-by-step instructions before you begin, so that you do not have to keep stopping to refer to the book. If you are receiving the massage, don't have a large meal beforehand, because the body will be working too hard digesting the food to be sufficiently relaxed.

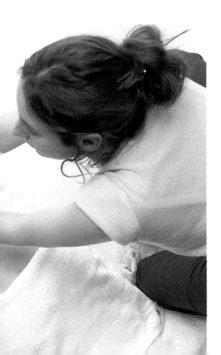

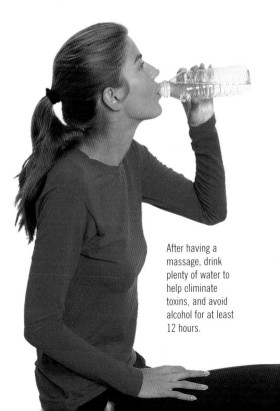

After having a massage, drink plenty of water to help eliminate toxins, and avoid alcohol for at least 12 hours.

Full back massage

▶ **1** Ask your partner to lie face down and place your hands on either side of the base of the spine. Using effleurage strokes (see page 64), glide your palms up the back to the neck. Continue over the shoulders, then return down the sides. Repeat several times.

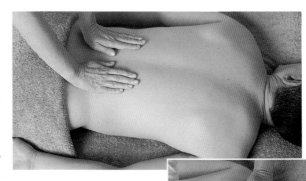

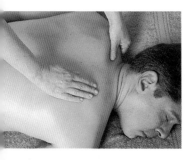

▲ **2** Knead the neck muscles by picking up the flesh and moving it away from the bone with a squeezing action. Neck muscles are often very tense, so try to be sensitive to how your partner feels.

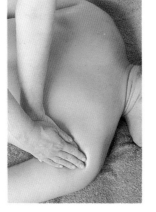

▲ **3** The next two steps describe a figure-eight movement, in which you should use the weight of your body to iron out tension. Start by putting one hand on top of the other at the neck. Move your hands diagonally across the back to go around one shoulder blade, then return to the center. Repeat around the other shoulder. Repeat several times.

▲ **4** Separate your hands and do figure-eight movements over the whole surface of the back. Remember to use your body weight to iron out tension.

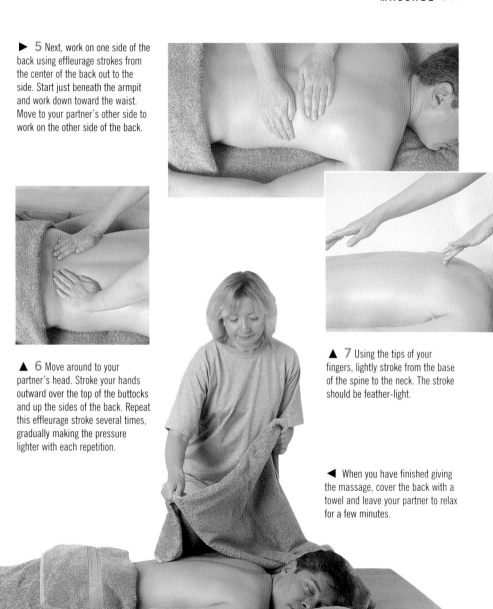

▶ **5** Next, work on one side of the back using effleurage strokes from the center of the back out to the side. Start just beneath the armpit and work down toward the waist. Move to your partner's other side to work on the other side of the back.

▲ **6** Move around to your partner's head. Stroke your hands outward over the top of the buttocks and up the sides of the back. Repeat this effleurage stroke several times, gradually making the pressure lighter with each repetition.

▲ **7** Using the tips of your fingers, lightly stroke from the base of the spine to the neck. The stroke should be feather-light.

◀ When you have finished giving the massage, cover the back with a towel and leave your partner to relax for a few minutes.

Lower back massage

▶ 1 Ask your partner to lie face down. Place one hand on each side of the spine, just above the buttocks and with your fingers pointing toward the head. Using long effleurage strokes (see page 64), work toward the head with both hands at the same time. Repeat several times.

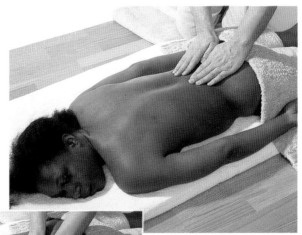

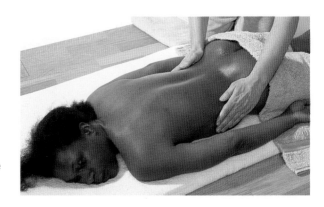

◀ 2 Keep your hands close to the spine and make sure the whole of the palms stays in contact with the back. Effleurage upward until your hands reach the lower ribcage, then turn your fingers outward and stroke your hands toward the sides.

▶ 3 Keeping your hands in this position, effleurage down the sides of the back toward the buttocks, reducing the pressure as you go. When your hands reach the buttocks, move them toward each other until the heels of your hands meet in the center, then rotate your fingers to point toward the head. Repeat these steps 2 and 3 until the back is thoroughly warmed up.

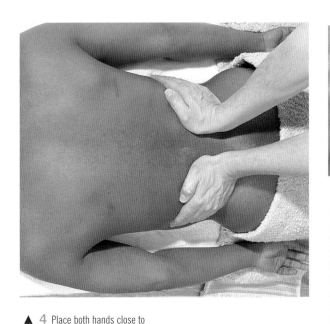

▲ 5 Apply pressure with the heel of the hand as you effleurage outward. Ease off the pressure as your fingertips touch the surface on which your partner is lying, and as the heel of the hand passes over the softer tissues. Return to the starting position and repeat several times. To finish, cover the back with a towel and leave your partner to relax for a few minutes.

▲ 4 Place both hands close to the spine with your fingers pointing outward, and the whole of your palms and fingers in contact with the back. Your hands should follow the curve of your partner's body.

◄ When massaging the lower back, avoid applying too much pressure to the kidney area, which lies just above the waistline.

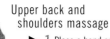

Upper back and shoulders massage

▶ 1 Place a hand on each side of the spine in the middle of the back, with your fingers pointing toward the head. Stroke toward the shoulders using effleurage (see page 64).

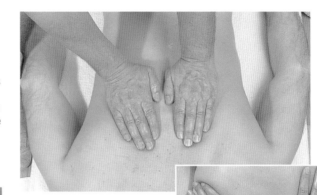

◀ 2 Move your hands out over the shoulders, keeping the pressure even. Effleurage around the shoulders, cupping your hands as you do so.

◀ 3 Ease off the pressure and effleurage down the sides of the back. Turn the heel of your hands toward the spine and move them to the middle of the back. Turn your fingers so that they are pointing toward the head once again and repeat steps 1–3 several times.

▲ 4 Position yourself at the head of your partner. Place your hands on the upper back, with both thumbs to one side of the spine. Press alternate thumbs into the muscles, working in the direction of the feet. Your thumbs will slide downward a short distance as you apply pressure. Repeat several times on both sides of the spine.

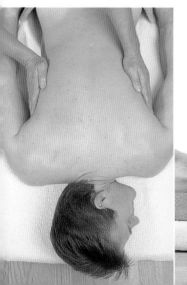

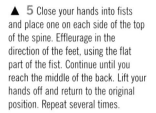

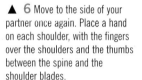

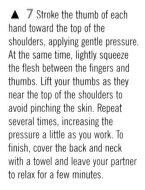

▲ **5** Close your hands into fists and place one on each side of the top of the spine. Effleurage in the direction of the feet, using the flat part of the fist. Continue until you reach the middle of the back. Lift your hands off and return to the original position. Repeat several times.

▲ **6** Move to the side of your partner once again. Place a hand on each shoulder, with the fingers over the shoulders and the thumbs between the spine and the shoulder blades.

▲ **7** Stroke the thumb of each hand toward the top of the shoulders, applying gentle pressure. At the same time, lightly squeeze the flesh between the fingers and thumbs. Lift your thumbs as they near the top of the shoulders to avoid pinching the skin. Repeat several times, increasing the pressure a little as you work. To finish, cover the back and neck with a towel and leave your partner to relax for a few minutes.

◄ When massaging with your fists, make sure that you use only the flat part of the fist, not the knuckles.

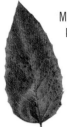

Massage during pregnancy

▶ 1 Ask your partner to sit upright, leaning on a table or the back of a chair. Place a hand on each side of the spine on the lower back with your fingers pointing toward the head. Using effleurage strokes (see page 64), work up toward the head, maintaining an even pressure.

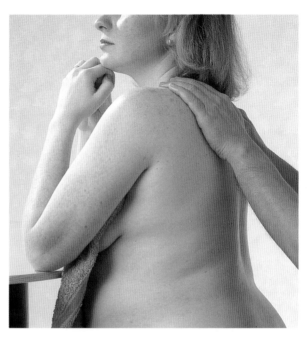

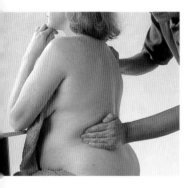

▲ 2 Place your hand to one side of the spine at the lower back. Applying even pressure with the heel of your hand, stroke out toward the side of the body. The stroke should be short, with most of the pressure on the muscles alongside the spine. Ease the pressure if you go over the kidney area, located just above the waistline. Repeat on the other side of the spine.

BASIC PRECAUTIONS

Massage can help to relieve the discomforts of pregnancy, but the following precautions should be taken.
- Avoid basil, fennel, juniper, rosemary, and sage aromatherapy oils. Instead, use camomile, geranium (in low doses), lavender, lemon, orange rose, and sandalwood essential oils
- Lying on the front can be uncomfortable after the fourth month of pregnancy, so lie on your side or sit up for back massages. If sitting, lean over the back of a chair or hold a towel-wrapped pillow for support
- Massage strokes should be applied more lightly than usual
- Rest quietly after the massage and get up slowly

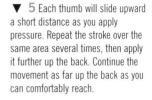

▼ **5** Each thumb will slide upward a short distance as you apply pressure. Repeat the stroke over the same area several times, then apply it further up the back. Continue the movement as far up the back as you can comfortably reach.

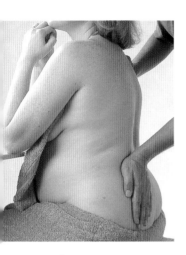

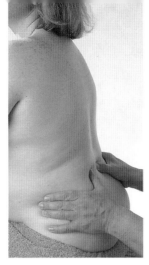

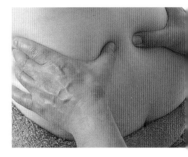

▲ **4** Kneel on the floor and place a hand on each side of the back, with your thumbs near the spine. Apply gentle pressure with your thumbs, starting as far down as you can comfortably reach.

▲ **3** Change direction and continue the movement downward, pointing your fingers toward the floor. Work on each side of the spine alternately.

▼ Massage is a wonderful way to relieve backache during pregnancy, as long as a few simple rules are followed (see box opposite).

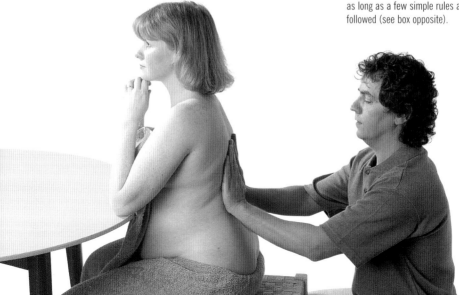

SELF-MASSAGE

If there is no one around to give you a massage when you need one, don't panic. You can massage yourself very easily and effectively. Most of us massage our shoulders from time to time to release tension, but you can also use your thumbs to massage those harder to reach areas along the sides of your spine, around your hipbones, and down your sacrum. Ideally, you should perform the lower back self-massage kneeling down, but if this is not possible, sit on a comfortable, backless stool.

Upper back self-massage

▶ **1** Place one hand over the opposite shoulder so that your fingers lie to the side of the spine. Press in a line down the side of the spine as far as you can comfortably reach. Move your fingers outward a little and repeat. Continue until you have reached the outer edge of your shoulder blade.

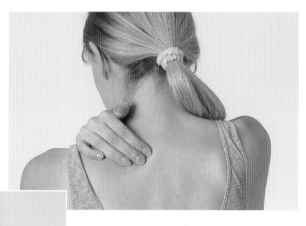

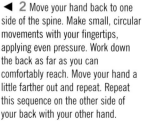

◀ **2** Move your hand back to one side of the spine. Make small, circular movements with your fingertips, applying even pressure. Work down the back as far as you can comfortably reach. Move your hand a little farther out and repeat. Repeat this sequence on the other side of your back with your other hand.

Lower back self-massage

▶ **1** Reach behind your back and place a thumb on each side of your spine, as high as you can comfortably reach. Press your thumbs in lines down both sides of your spine, keeping them level. Move your thumbs a little farther apart and repeat, continuing in this way until you have covered the whole of your lower back with vertical lines of pressure.

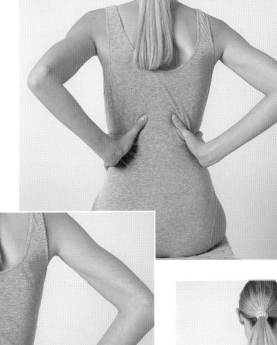

▲ **2** Place your hands on your hips so that your thumbs rest on the bony ridge of your hipbones. Press into the soft tissue just above your hipbones, working outward from the center and angling your thumbs slightly downward so that they reach under the bone. Work out to each side of the hips.

▶ **3** Keep your hands on your hips and move your thumbs to either side of your spine. Move them down onto the flat triangle of bone at the base of your spine (the sacrum). Press down the sacrum with the tips of your thumbs. Slide your palms farther down the sides of your hips as you press lower.

ACUPRESSURE

Acupressure is an ancient Far Eastern massage technique that stimulates the flow of essential body energy, known as Qi or Chi, at key points along the body's energy channels, known as meridians. Acupressure works in the same way as acupuncture, but finger pressure is used to stimulate the relevant points rather than needles. Acupressure can be used to relieve common symptoms and ailments, including the build-up of tension in the back.

Full back routine

▶ 1 Ask your partner to lie face down. Place one hand at the top of the back on one side of the spine. Place your other hand a little farther down, on the same side. Lean your body weight onto your hands. Do not apply pressure to the spine itself. Keeping the pressure on the upper hand steady, release the lower hand and move it a little farther down the back. Lean onto it again. Repeat this process all the way down the spine, to just below waist level. You may need to move your upper hand farther down the spine as you work your way down.

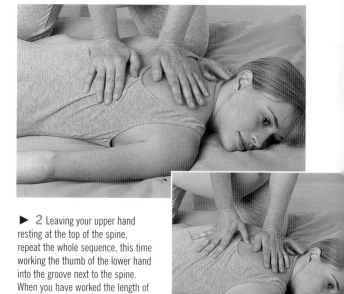

▶ 2 Leaving your upper hand resting at the top of the spine, repeat the whole sequence, this time working the thumb of the lower hand into the groove next to the spine. When you have worked the length of the spine, change sides and work down the opposite side of the spine in the same way, using the flat of the hand and then the thumb.

Lower back routine

▶ 1 Use your fingertips to find the flat bony triangle at the base of the spine (the sacrum). Place a thumb on each side of the sacrum and gradually lean your body weight onto your thumbs.

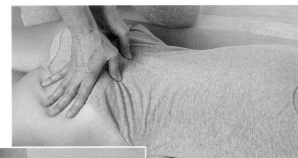

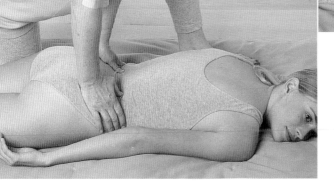

◀ 2 Place your hands on top of your partner's hipbones, with your fingers out to the side and your thumbs on either side of the spine, a little below waist level. Apply pressure at this point. Gradually move your thumbs outward over the curve of the hipbones, applying pressure at regular intervals.

PRESSURE POINTS FOR THE BACK

You can apply acupressure to key points on your own body whenever you experience back pain. Simply find the relevant point, then apply gentle, continuous pressure with your thumb or forefinger for a few minutes.

- For intense lower back pain: in the middle of the fold behind either knee (but not if you have varicose veins there)
- For mid- to lower back pain: on the back of your right hand, where the bones meet between the fourth and fifth digits

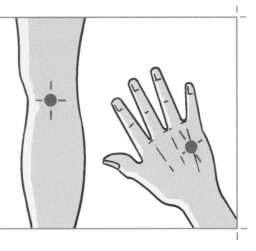

HYDROTHERAPY

Every time you take a bath or shower, you are having hydrotherapy, which simply means any type of treatment using water. As well as a relaxing warm bath, you can try saunas, steam baths, whirlpool baths, and sitz baths to help soothe an aching back and ease tension. The warm water helps to relax muscles and opens up blood vessels to improve circulation, while the pressurized jets of a whirlpool bath give you a massage while you soak.

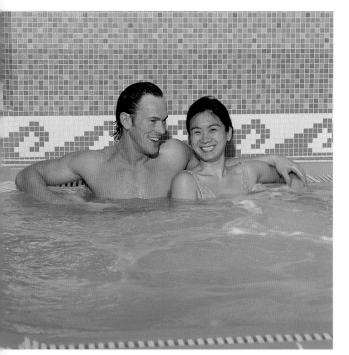

Whirlpool baths

Whirlpool baths gently massage aching muscles and help to soothe inflammation of surrounding tissues. You can visit a health club or spa to have a whirlpool bath, but if you have a shower head with a flexible hose, you can try something similar at home by directing a jet of water onto the affected area of your back.

Sitz baths

Sit in a shallow hot bath with your feet in a bowl of cold water for a few minutes, then reverse the process, sitting in a cold bath with your feet in hot water. Massage your hips and abdomen while you bathe.

Saunas

The intense dry heat of a sauna soothes aching muscles and joints, speeds up the metabolism, boosts the immune system, and clears the skin of impurities. Stay in the sauna for 5–10 minutes at a time, taking a cool shower in between sessions. Drink plenty of water before, during, and after a sauna to prevent dehydration, and don't eat immediately beforehand. Saunas often have two levels of benches – start on a lower one, where it is cooler, then move to the higher bench when you are used to the heat.

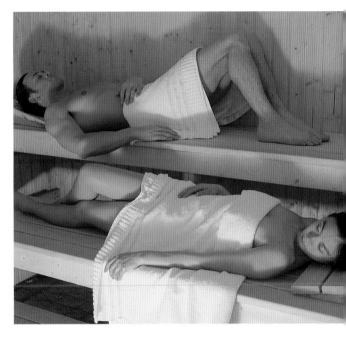

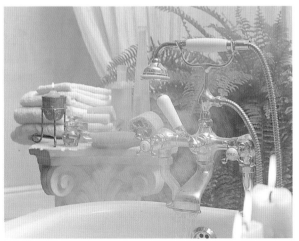

Steam baths

The moist heat of a steam bath is also good for an aching back. You can visit a gym or spa, or create your own steam room at home. Close the bathroom doors and windows, then switch on the shower or faucet at its highest temperature until the room fills with steam. Relax in the room for up to 20 minutes, then have a warm shower, followed by a quick burst under a cold shower afterwards.

HERBAL **HEALING**

Herbal therapy has been used for thousands of years to combat pain and promote good health. Herbal baths combine the medicinal properties of herbs with the benefits of heat to soothe and relieve tension, and impart a wonderful sense of well-being. Another way to provide relief from back pain is by applying compresses alternately soaked in hot and cold water; the benefits can be increased by using water in which herbs have been steeped. The heat from the hot compress opens up the blood vessels and relaxes the muscles; the cold compress then restricts the blood vessels, reducing blood flow from the inflamed area.

Herbal baths

Make an infusion by steeping a handful of fresh or dried herbs in boiling water for 15–20 minutes. Strain the liquid and add it to your bath water. Alternatively, tie the herbs inside a small square of cheesecloth and hang the herbal pouch under the faucet, so that the water runs through the herbs and into your bath. Add some oatmeal to the pouch of herbs to soften the water and moisturize dry skin.

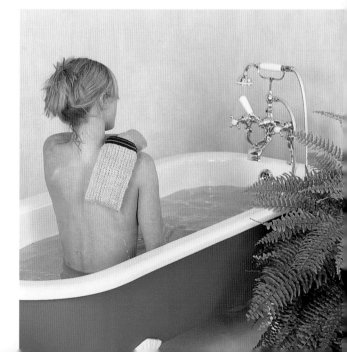

Enhance your herbal bath by rubbing your shoulders and back with a sisal back scrubber.

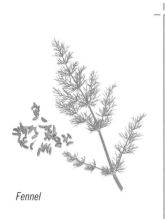

Fennel

HERBS FOR
STIMULATION

Herbs that are good for
refreshing and stimulating
the mind and body include:
• basil
• bay
• fennel
• ginger
• pine
• rosemary
• thyme

HERBS FOR
RELAXATION

Herbs that are good for
relaxing tense muscles and
relieving anxiety include:
• catnip
• camomile
• lavender

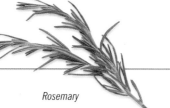

Hot and cold compresses

Rosemary

You will need two cloths or towels (large enough to cover the
painful area when folded over two or three times) and some hot
and cold water (from the faucet will be fine). For added benefit,
make herbal infusions in the same way as for a herbal bath, then
heat some of the strained infusion, cool the remainder, and use
these in place of plain water. Soak the first cloth in hot water, then
wring it out. Lay the cloth onto the affected area and leave for
about three minutes. Repeat with the second cloth using cold
water, leaving it in place for about a minute.

Repeat both hot and cold stages,
continuing for about 20 minutes.
If the pain is in your lower
back, you will probably be
able to apply the
compresses yourself.
If the pain is higher
up, ask a friend or
partner to apply
them while you
lie face down.

Hot and cold compresses are an
effective way to relieve both chronic
and acute back pain. Make
compresses by soaking cloths in
water or a herbal infusion.
Alternatively, use an ice pack and
a hot-water bottle.

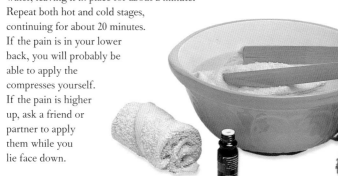

BACK **BEAUTIFUL**

As well as keeping your back healthy, it is important to pamper your skin to keep it soft and supple. Apply an exfoliating cream with a stiff back scrubber, such as a sisal mitt or loofah, to invigorate the skin, improve the circulation, and remove dead skin cells. Exfoliate about once a week when you are in the bath or shower. Massage moisturizer all over your back every day.

SOAP

Choose a soap that has been specially designed for the type of skin you have.
- Dry skin: soaps containing almond, jojoba, avocado, and olive oils
- Oily skin: soaps containing citrus or fruit oils
- Sensitive skin: vegetable-based or glycerine soaps containing aloe vera and vitamin E

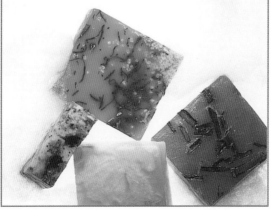

Body moisturizers

Apply moisturizer every day after you have a bath or shower. Heavy creams contain more oil than water, have a richer texture than lotions and gels, and are best suited to dry skins. Gels are made from natural emollient resins and gums rather than oils, and are suitable for normal to oily skin. If you choose a moisturizer made from natural ingredients, use it within 3–6 months. Other types of moisturizer will keep for about 12–18 months. Always throw moisturizer away if it changes color, looks cloudy, or you notice that it starts to smell differently to normal.

Exfoliators

Products containing abrasive ingredients, such as tiny pieces of crushed nut kernels, rice grains, and oatmeal, work by gently rubbing away dead skin cells. Gently massage a little into the skin, then wash it off with warm water. You can use some products straight from the container; others need to be mixed with a little water in the palm of the hand before use. For maximum effect, use exfoliation creams with back scrubbers, such as loofahs, sisal mitts, and bristle brushes, to improve circulation, get rid of dead skin cells, and unclog blocked pores. Exfoliate about once a week.

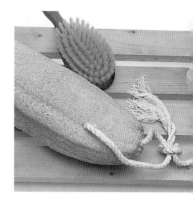

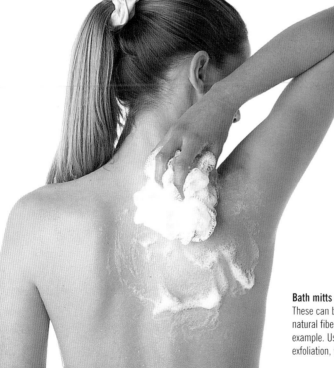

Brushes and loofahs
Long-handled back brushes should be used wet if the bristles are stiff, but can be used either wet or dry if the bristles are soft enough. Check by rubbing your hand against them. Loofahs are made from the natural fibers of the dishcloth gourd (*Luffa*) and should be used wet. Use a long loofah to reach all areas of your back.

Bath mitts and scrubbers
These can be made from artificial or natural fibers – nylon or sisal, for example. Use them dry for maximum exfoliation, wet for a gentler effect.

BACK **PACKS**

You can apply a face pack to your face, so why not treat your back to a back pack, using simple recipes and natural ingredients. For maximum benefit, apply a back pack at least once every two weeks.

Strawberry smoother

Use this pack to exfoliate the skin. This will allow the skin to absorb more moisture, and so make it softer.

Mud pack

Mud is a rich source of minerals, which can help to relax and revitalize an aching back.

You will need

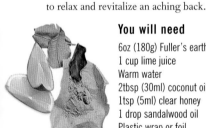

6oz (180g) Fuller's earth powder
1 cup lime juice
Warm water
2tbsp (30ml) coconut oil
1tsp (5ml) clear honey
1 drop sandalwood oil
Plastic wrap or foil

Mix the Fuller's earth powder and lime juice together to make a thick paste. Add a little warm water and stir until creamy. Stir in the coconut oil, honey, and sandalwood oil. Spread the mud pack over your back and cover with plastic wrap or foil to retain the heat generated by the pack. After about 20 minutes, have a warm shower. Drink some water afterwards to prevent dehydration.

You will need

6 cups fresh, crushed strawberries
12tbsp (180ml) live, plain yogurt
3tbsp (45ml) cornstarch
3tbsp (45ml) clear honey
½ cup oatmeal flakes
½tsp (2.5ml) lavender oil

Mix all of the ingredients into a paste. Spread it on your back and relax for 15–20 minutes. Rinse off with a warm shower.

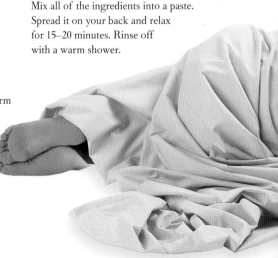

Pepper pack

This pack is good for a painful back, because it helps to bring blood to the surface of the skin and increase circulation.

You will need

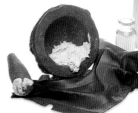

1tbsp (15ml) cayenne
    pepper powder
8tbsp (120ml) cornstarch
Warm water
Thick cloth or towel
Hot-water bottle or radiator

Mix the cayenne pepper and cornstarch with sufficient water to make a creamy paste. Spread the mixture onto a folded cloth or towel, fold it again, and place it on a hot-water bottle or radiator to heat up. Apply the cloth to the painful area and keep it there for about 15 minutes. Rinse off with warm water.

Seaweed wrap

Seaweed is packed with nutrients, which stimulate circulation and soothe muscular aches.

You will need

6oz (180g) concentrated,
    dried, micronized seaweed
    (available from health
    food/Japanese stores)
Warm water
2tbsp (30ml) almond oil
2 drops rosemary oil
Plastic wrap or foil

Mix the dried seaweed with a little warm water, then stir in the almond and rosemary oils to make a thick paste. Spread the mixture on your back and cover with foil or plastic wrap to retain the heat. Have a warm shower after 20–30 minutes. Drink some water afterwards to prevent dehydration.

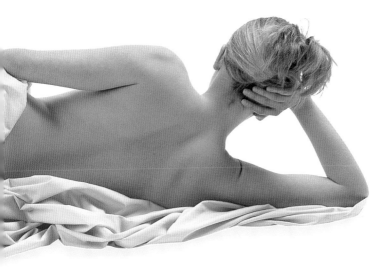

Although many of us apply face packs to give our skin a healthy glow, and smooth rich moisturizing creams onto our arms and legs, we often neglect our backs – probably because it is more difficult to reach and is out of view. Try using these simple, natural recipes to pamper your skin and make your back beautiful.

SKIN CARE

It is particularly important to follow a sensible skin care routine if you suffer from problems such as spots. Choosing the right washing product can make a world of difference. Some herbal remedies are particularly effective for inflamed or irritated skin. The skin can also suffer during the summer months, especially in hot climates. Never go out in the sun without first applying sun cream, and be especially careful around 11am–3pm when the sun is at its strongest.

Skin care in the sun

Shoulders are particularly prone to sunburn. Always apply sun cream with a sun protection factor of at least SPF 15 if you are going outside with your back or shoulders exposed. Remember that you can get sunburn even on a cloudy day. Apply cream regularly and always after swimming.

Spots

It is not uncommon to have spots on the shoulders or upper back, even after puberty. If you do have any spots, resist the temptation to squeeze them. Keep the area clean, but do not overwash – you will only remove surface oil. Use a hypo-allergenic soap or cleansing cream (or a soap specially designed for a baby's delicate skin) no more than twice a day.

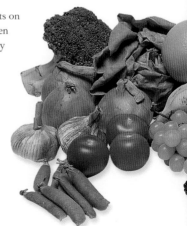

IRRITATED OR INFLAMED SKIN

To sooth inflamed or irritated skin, apply ointments or compresses (see page 81) containing the following herbs:
- red clover
- borage
- burdock root
- chickweed
- comfrey
- marigold (calendula)

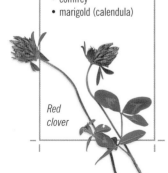

Red clover

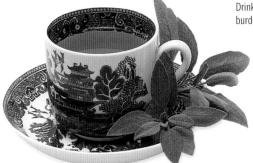

Herbal tea

Drinking a herbal tea made from burdock, dandelion, echinacea, and yellow dock leaves may help to clear spots.

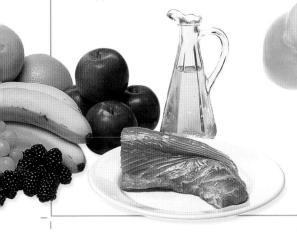

EATING FOR HEALTHY SKIN

Eating a balanced diet is the best way to healthy skin. Try to eat foods containing some of the following nutrients each week and your skin will benefit:

- vitamins A, B-complex, and E
- fish oils (from oily fish such as mackerel and sardines)
- zinc (oysters are a rich source)
- selenium and magnesium supplements
- evening primrose oil

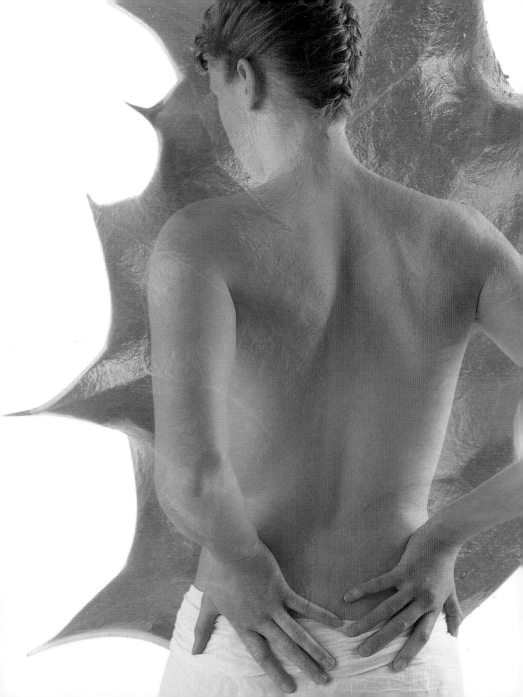

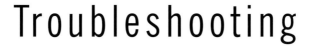

Troubleshooting

IF YOUR
BACKACHE DOES
NOT GO AWAY AFTER
REST AND RELAXATION,
YOU NEED TO SEEK
PROFESSIONAL HELP. THIS
CHAPTER TELLS YOU WHAT
TO DO IF THE PAIN IS
ACUTE, WHEN YOU SHOULD
SEE A DOCTOR, AND HOW
SOME COMPLEMENTARY
TREATMENTS CAN HELP
WITH CHRONIC AND
ACUTE BACK PAIN.

WHEN TO **SEE A DOCTOR**

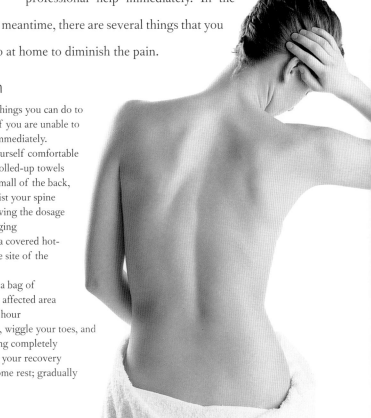

Rest and relaxation may be enough to treat many cases of backache, but in some instances, such as the first attack of acute back pain or when the pain lasts for more than two or three days, it is sensible to seek further help. If the pain is so severe that you cannot move, seek professional help immediately. In the meantime, there are several things that you can do at home to diminish the pain.

Acute back pain

There are a number of things you can do to relieve acute back pain if you are unable to seek professional help immediately.

- Lie down and make yourself comfortable with small pillows or rolled-up towels under your neck, the small of the back, or knees; try not to twist your spine
- Take painkillers, following the dosage guidance on the packaging
- For muscle pain, hold a covered hot-water bottle against the site of the pain to bring relief
- For skeletal pain, hold a bag of crushed ice against the affected area for five minutes every hour
- Try to move your legs, wiggle your toes, and bend your knees – being completely immobile will prolong your recovery
- Try to relax and get some rest; gradually the pain should lessen

What a doctor may do

The doctor will examine you and ask questions about the pain – what brought it on, what it feels like, and where exactly it occurs. She or he may also arrange for blood tests or X-rays to be carried out, to find out what is causing the pain and decide what treatment you may need. In the meantime, you may be prescribed painkillers, anti-inflammatory drugs, and muscle relaxants and be advised to stay in bed.

Complementary therapies

Therapies such as osteopathy, chiropractic, physiotherapy, acupuncture, and Alexander technique can help to relieve pain and treat its underlying causes. Always make sure that you consult a fully qualified practitioner. Ask a friend or a doctor for a recommendation. Alternatively, seek out a natural health center in your area, or contact a national organization that maintains a listing of therapists and teachers.

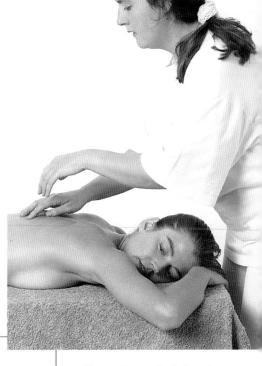

Massage is extremely relaxing and soothing, and can provide instant relief from back pain.

WARNING
Take note of any symptoms accompanying your back pain and seek urgent medical advice if:
- you notice any numbness or pins and needles in one or both legs
- your bladder or bowel habits alter in any way
- you feel weak, giddy, or nauseous for no apparent reason
- you also have pain elsewhere in your body
- you feel generally tired and unwell, have lost your appetite, or have lost weight recently
- the pain gets progressively worse and is not helped by changing your position

OSTEOPATHY

In osteopathy (which means "bone treatment"), the bones, joints, muscles, ligaments, and connective tissues are manipulated by the osteopath to help both chronic and acute back pain, often succeeding where conventional treatment has failed. Osteopathy is based on the premise that the functioning of the body will be impaired if the stucture is out of alignment. Trained in anatomy and physiology, osteopaths are able to recognize and correct problems using a wide variety of techniques.

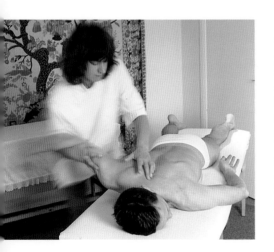

Osteopathy involves a wide variety of treatments, from gentle stretching and manipulation to articulation and dramatic high-velocity thrusts.

Diagnosis

You will be asked about your medical history, in particular back problems, but also about any other aches and pains. You will also be questioned about your lifestyle and emotional health, because the backache may be caused by something you do in your everyday life, such as sitting hunched over a desk for long periods. You will be asked to take off some clothes and stand, sit, or lie on a treatment table while the osteopath examines your joints, tendons, and ligaments. She or he will take you through a series of movements to see how you move and may test your reflexes. In the United States, osteopaths are also doctors and may send you for X-rays, blood tests, and other diagnostic tests; elsewhere, they will refer you to a doctor to have these tests carried out if necessary.

Many people experience relief from back pain and an improvement in the health of their back after a single treatment, but you will probably need around 3–6 sessions with an osteopath for maximum benefit.

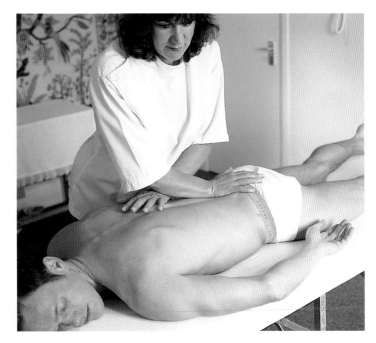

Treatment

If osteopathy is appropriate, the osteopath will draw up an individual treatment program. Typically, this would include:
- massage for relaxing stiff muscles
- stretching spinal joints (traction) to help with mobility
- manipulation, where the osteopath manually moves your body to separate the spinal vertebrae gently
- quick, high-velocity thrusts to a joint to restore movement; these may make a clicking sound, but are not painful (there are alternative methods should you prefer not to be "clicked")
- light touch and positioning of the body to reduce tension and restore balance
- passive movements of the back
- gentle exercises
- advice on lifestyle, such as exercise, smoking, drinking, and diet

Results

You will probably feel more mobile immediately after the treatment. If there is inflammation, however, this needs to settle before you will get relief from the pain. It is not unusual for a patient to feel worse for a day or so while the body adjusts to the realignments. The number of treatments you need will depend on your individual situation – most people get maximum benefit from 3–6 sessions.

CHIROPRACTIC

The word chiropractic has Greek origins and means "manual practice." The theory behind chiropractic is that if any of the spinal vertebrae moves out of position, it can affect the surrounding nerves, muscles, and ligaments. Chiropractors use their hands to manipulate the joints and muscles in the back and restore normal function. The main difference between chiropractic and osteopathy is that osteopaths consider the main effect of their treatment to be on the blood supply, while chiropractors believe the nerves are the important element.

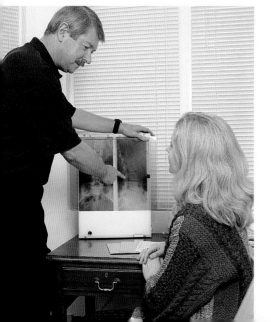

Diagnosis

At the first consultation, you will be asked detailed questions about your medical history, your lifestyle, and the back problems you are having. The chiropractor will examine you and watch how you walk, stand, and sit. She or he will carry out various tests – such as moving your body from side to side, sliding your arms down your legs, or lifting your legs – to see how these movements affect your spine. X-rays may also be taken as part of the diagnosis.

Chiropractors look very carefully at X-rays of the spine to assess even very slight changes to the angles of the vertebrae.

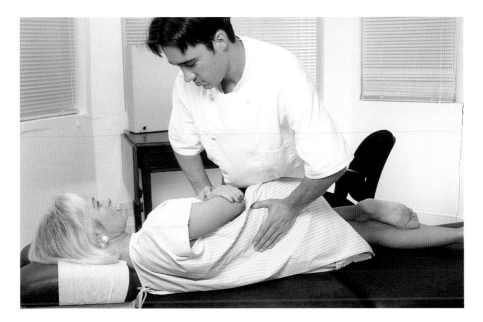

Treatment

During a treatment session, you will be asked either to sit or lie on a chiropractic table, wearing underwear or a modesty gown. The chiropractor will use various techniques to stretch and relax the muscles and to "unlock" the joints. The most well-known chiropractic technique is the high-velocity thrust, which is also used by osteopaths (see pages 92–93). This involves the chiropractor pushing the relevant spinal joint as far as it can go, then quickly thrusting on the vertebrae, to take it even further. The joint may make a loud cracking sound when this happens. This can sound alarming, but don't worry, the noise is caused by the facet joints moving apart slightly, not by cracking bone. Unless your back pain is so

Chiropractors employ about 50 different ways to adjust the spine, but most use only 15 routinely.

severe that it hurts even to be touched, chiropractic techniques are not painful, though they can feel a little strange.

Results

Many people feel immediately better, and even revitalized, after treatment. Some people experience a little stiffness afterwards. This is perfectly normal and will pass within a day or so. The number of sessions you need will depend on your individual problem – some people require only one or two, while others need treatment over a number of months.

PHYSIOTHERAPY

Physiotherapists – also known as physical therapists – use physical techniques to help cure back pain and stiffness, and to restore the back's full range of movement, often after injury. The techniques include manipulation, massage, exercise, and heat treatments as well as the use of electrical equipment and traction apparatus. Physiotherapy helps to relax tense muscles, strengthen weakened muscles, improve circulation to speed up the healing process, and reduce inflammation. Some electrical treatments alter the way the nervous system perceives pain.

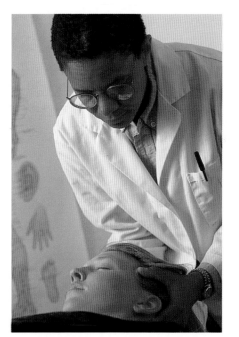

Diagnosis, treatment, results

The physiotherapist will take a full history of your back problem, ask you to carry out some simple tests, such as taking off your jacket, to see how mobile you are, and examine your back. This will help the therapist to devise an appropriate treatment program for you and your particular problem, which may combine several physical techniques as well as advice on posture and how to carry out everyday activities without harming your back. You will probably be given exercises to do at home. Some patients may benefit immediately and require only one or two sessions; others will need a course of treatment over several months.

A physiotherapist may employ mobilization, which involves passive movements of the affected area. This helps to relieve pain and increase the patient's mobility.

Physical techniques

Physiotherapists use a number of physical techniques to treat back pain, including:

Massage Massaging ligaments and muscles to relax them, increase the range of movement, and improve circulation.

Mobilization Gentle, passive, repetitive movements to relieve pain and increase the range of movement.

Exercise Strengthening the muscles is an important part of regaining mobility. You may be asked to carry out movements while the physiotherapist pushes against you, and exercise the muscles without moving the joint.

Electrotherapy There are three main types of electrotherapy.
- Ultrasound – high-frequency soundwaves are applied to injured muscles, tendons, or ligaments to relax muscular spasm, reduce swelling, and promote healing
- Interferential treatment – electrodes are attached to each side of the painful area and a mild electrical current passed between them, which blocks the body's natural pain receptors and can also be used to contract the muscles without exercising them
- TENS (transcutaneous electrical nerve stimulation) – mild electrical currents are used to override the body's perception of pain

Hydrotherapy Exercising in water to strengthen back muscles and improve mobility.

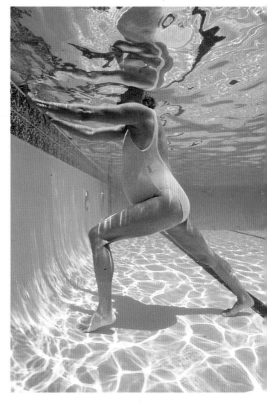

Hydrotherapy is particularly good for back pain, since the water supports the body's weight and relieves pressure on the spine. It is therefore highly suitable for pregnant women.

Hot and Cold Treatments Infrared lamps help to relax muscles; cold compresses can reduce inflammation.

Traction Stretches the spine by pulling the spinal joints apart, often using special apparatus.

ALEXANDER TECHNIQUE

The Alexander technique – developed by 19th-century Australian actor FM Alexander – can help to improve posture, alleviate backache, and prevent back problems from occurring. Practitioners prefer to be known as teachers rather than therapists. The Alexander technique is based on the idea that posture influences every area of our lives, both physically and mentally. It helps you to "unlearn" bad habits, relax tense muscles (especially in the neck and shoulders), and develop the posture that puts least stress on the spine.

Lying down

The Alexander technique teacher may start by asking you to lie down with knees bent and head raised. Here, the teacher is showing the patient how to relax so that her limbs remain in natural alignment.

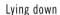

Diagnosis

You need to be taught the Alexander technique by a qualified teacher in a one-to-one session – we all have our own unique posture and need a program devised especially for us. The teacher may start by watching how you sit, stand, walk, and lie down, so that she or he can analyze your posture and how you use your body.

Treatment

Over a series of classes, the teacher will help you to become aware of your bad habits and to learn good ones by gently guiding your body into the correct positions and explaining what you should do. This may involve:

• asking you to lie down with your knees bent and your head raised,

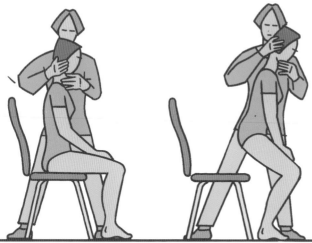

Standing up

A common postural problem when standing up is to pull the head back, rather than maintain the correct alignment of the head, neck, and back. Here, the Alexander technique teacher is guiding the position of the patient's head as she stands up.

then showing you how to relax so that your limbs are naturally aligned
- showing you how to stand up while keeping your spine straight, rather than leaning forward and moving your head and body as one
- showing you how to sit down with your back straight and head forward, then how to sit with the appropriate amount of curve in your back

Results

The course may last from six weeks up to a year, depending on your posture and progress. In addition to relieving backache, you will, over time, learn to use your body in a more efficient way, your breathing will be improved, and you will generally feel more confident and relaxed.

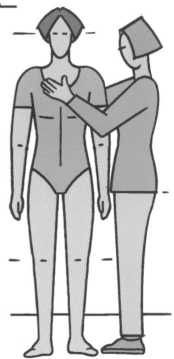

Standing

Once standing, the teacher guides the patient's spinal alignment to help her achieve a lengthened and more balanced posture.

ACUPUNCTURE

The ancient Oriental art of acupuncture uses fine needles to restore the body's natural harmony and relieve back pain. Acupuncturists believe that a life force, known as Qi or Chi (pronounced "chee"), passes through an invisible network of channels in the body (known as meridians). The flow of Qi is controlled by two energy forces, known as yin and yang. If the Qi is blocked or depleted, or the yin and yang are out of balance, ill health can occur. The flow of energy can be altered by stimulating key points along the meridians with fine needles.

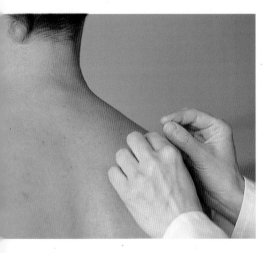

Once in place, acupuncture needles may be rotated between the finger and thumb to help release any blockages in the flow in Qi.

Diagnosis

The acupuncturist will ask you various questions, many of which may seem to have little to do with your back, in order to build up an overall picture of your health and energy flow. She or he will note your appearance, behavior, hair, and skin, how you speak and move, and will probably examine your tongue and check the six meridian pulses on each wrist.

Treatment

The acupuncturist will insert very fine, sterile, stainless steel needles into the places where the energies need to be changed. This may be your back, but sometimes your hands, arms, legs, abdomen, and head. This is because each organ in the body has a meridian, and it is by working at appropriate points along that meridian that the acupuncturist can improve the functioning of the

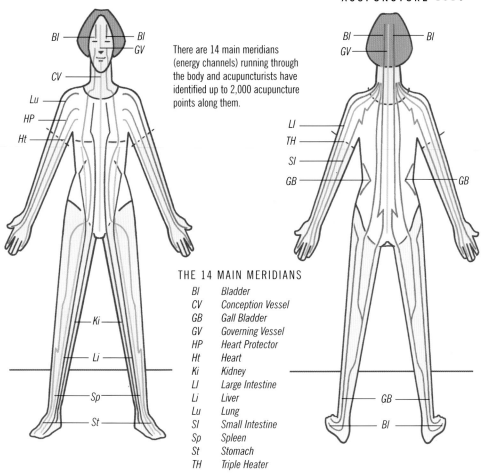

There are 14 main meridians (energy channels) running through the body and acupuncturists have identified up to 2,000 acupuncture points along them.

THE 14 MAIN MERIDIANS

BI	Bladder
CV	Conception Vessel
GB	Gall Bladder
GV	Governing Vessel
HP	Heart Protector
Ht	Heart
Ki	Kidney
LI	Large Intestine
Li	Liver
Lu	Lung
SI	Small Intestine
Sp	Spleen
St	Stomach
TH	Triple Heater

organ; treatment may therefore not be located at the precise point of the pain. The needles may be inserted just below the skin or deeper, depending on the location, and left in place for up to 30 minutes. Inserting the needles does not hurt, but you may feel a slight aching sensation when they are in place. This is a positive sign: it means that the needle has reached the right place and is affecting the flow of Qi.

Results

For many patients, acupuncture can produce a dramatic improvement after just one session, but it is more likely that you will need to have around 6–12 sessions to feel a real benefit.

EXERCISES FOR **MINOR BACK PROBLEMS**

We all suffer from minor back problems from time to time. These exercises have been devised to help rectify some of the most common ones, such as shoulder tension, a cricked neck, and an aching back after activities such as gardening and housework. The exercises can also be used preventively.

Shoulder tension

Tension in the shoulders and mid-back area is an extremely common problem, particularly for those whose work involves sitting at a desk or working at a computer screen all day. These two exercises will help to release tense muscles in the shoulders and back, and stretch the upper spine.

WARNING
If you experience acute pain, or have any doubts about the health of your back, consult a medical practitioner before embarking on any course of exercise.

Try to hold your shoulders back.

Keep your elbows in and palms pressed together.

Prayer pose
Stand with your palms behind your back and fingers pointing downward. Rotate your wrists so that your fingers point up your back. Draw your elbows back and press the heels of your hands together. Hold for between 30 seconds and two minutes.

Stand straight with your feet a few inches apart.

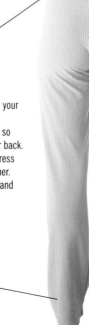

Figure-eight

Sitting down, clasp your fingers behind your neck with your elbows touching. Round your back as much possible. Draw a large figure-eight in the air with your elbows, so that you feel the stretch in your mid-back. Repeat several times.

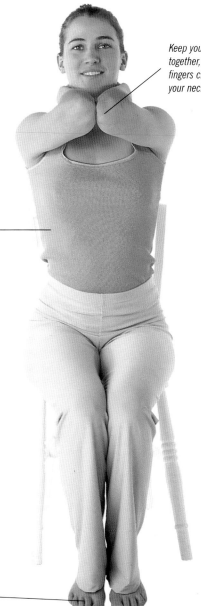

Keep your elbows together, with your fingers clasped behind your neck.

Sit up straight in the chair.

DO
- keep the spine upright

DON'T
- allow your lower back to compress

GOOD FOR
- releasing tension in the shoulders
- easing strain in the mid-back

Keep your feet together.

Lower back strain

This exercise is particularly good for stretching the lower back after gardening, housework, or other similar activities. Stand with feet apart and toes turned slightly outward. Bend your knees and squat, trying to keep your heels on the floor. Adjust your feet sidewise if necessary. Initially, you may find it easier to hold onto a support, such as the edge of a chair seat. Hold the position for at least one minute, gradually increasing to three minutes.

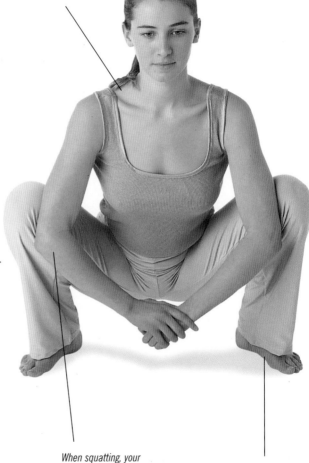

Keep your back straight.

DO
- practice the exercise — it will become easier over time

DON'T
- overbalance — hold onto a chair or other support to steady yourself if necessary

GOOD FOR
- stretching the lower back

When squatting, your elbows should be inside your knees.

Try to keep your feet flat on the floor.

Period pain

This exercise is a highly effective remedy for period pain in the abdominal and lower back area. Sit with the soles of your feet together, pulling your heels into the pubic bone. Breathe in, then as you breathe out, push your knees to the floor, clasping your feet with your hands. Bend forward, lowering your head toward your toes. Hold the pose for one minute.

▼ 1 Sit upright on the floor and hold the soles of your feet together.

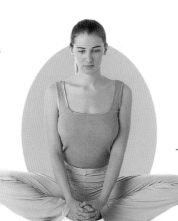

DO
- take your time
- keep breathing

DON'T
- force yourself to go lower than is comfortable

GOOD FOR
- easing stomach pains
- improving blood supply to the uterus

▶ 2 Bend forward, keeping your back as straight as possible.

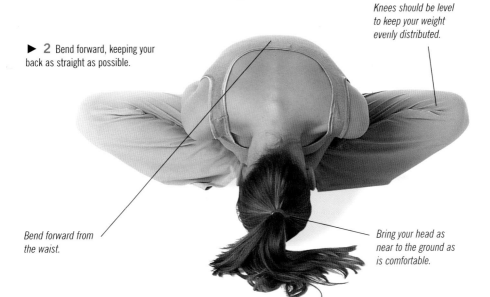

Knees should be level to keep your weight evenly distributed.

Bend forward from the waist.

Bring your head as near to the ground as is comfortable.

Cricked neck

Almost everyone has experienced waking up with a sore neck after sleeping in an awkward position. This exercise will help to relieve the pain of a cricked neck. In a seated position, put your right hand on your right shoulder, and your left hand on top of your head. Using the weight of your hands, tilt your head to the left while gently pulling down on the right shoulder. Breathe in. Breathing out, feel the muscles slacken a little. Do five inhalation/exhalation cycles in total, then repeat the process on the other side.

Gently pull on the shoulder with your hand.

DO
• allow your body to relax as you breathe in and out

DON'T
• pull too hard on the shoulder

GOOD FOR
• easing neck stiffness
• relaxing taut muscles and ligaments

Working in pairs

If someone has a very stiff neck, it may be easier to work in pairs. To perform this exercise on a partner, standing behind the chair, put one hand on the shoulder and your other hand on the head. As before, gently pull down on the shoulder and tilt the head in the opposite direction. Repeat on the other side.

*Use your other hand to
tilt your head in the
opposite direction.*

*Rest your foot in the
crook of your elbow.*

Sciatica

This exercise is good for
relieving buttock and thigh
pain, such as sciatica. Sitting
in a chair, lift up your left leg.
Place your left foot into the
crook of your right elbow.
Swing your left arm around
your left knee and join hands,
as if you were cradling a baby.
Sit up straight and feel the
stretch through the buttocks.
Hold for between 30 seconds
and one minute. Repeat on the
other side.

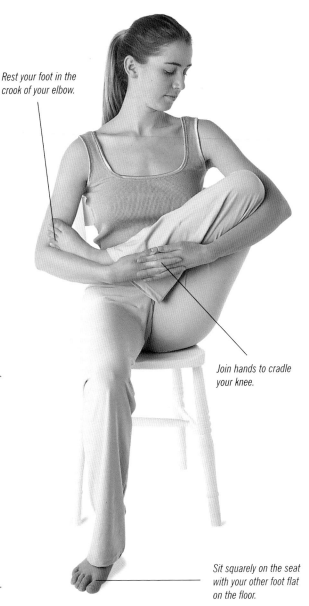

*Join hands to cradle
your knee.*

DO
- sit up straight to feel
  the stretch in your
  buttocks

DON'T
- forget to work on both
  sides, even if the pain
  is more severe on one
  side than the other

GOOD FOR
- buttock and thigh pain

*Sit squarely on the seat
with your other foot flat
on the floor.*

General stiffness

This exercise helps to banish stiffness from the whole back. You will need something solid to suspend your weight from – a doorframe will do. Stand in front of the support and grip your fingers around it. Bend your knees until you feel the stretch through the whole spine, reaching down to the lower back and pelvis. Hold your balance on the balls of your feet and breathe normally. Hold the pose for 30 seconds to one minute.

DO
- feel the stretch through the length of your spine

DON'T
- position your hands too close together
- raise your shoulders

GOOD FOR
- general back stiffness
- stretching the whole spine

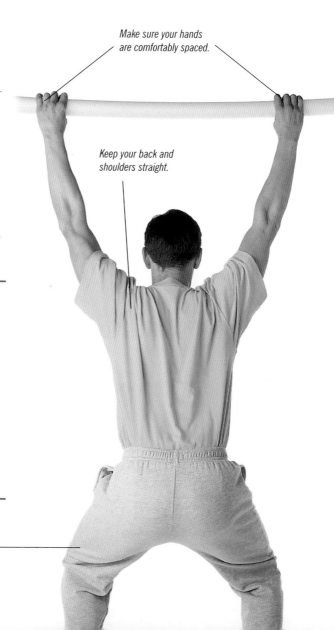

Make sure your hands are comfortably spaced.

Keep your back and shoulders straight.

Bend your knees as you clasp the support.

SPECIFIC **BACK PROBLEMS**

While much back pain is caused by strain or poor posture, it can also be

the result of a specific condition. The diagnosis of such back problems

must be made by a qualified medical practitioner, and self-help measures

should not be undertaken unless recommended by the practitioner.

Ankylosing spondylitis

Inflammation of the joints between the spinal vertebrae. Disks and ligaments calcify and "lock" together, making the spine increasingly stiff and sometimes hunched.

Coccydynia

Pain around the coccyx (tailbone), often caused by a fall.

Fibrositis

Pain and stiffness of the muscles, which may be caused by prolonged tension.

Infections

Kidney and viral infections, such as flu, can also cause back pain. Accompanying symptoms may include a temperature of 100°F (38°C) or above, diarrhea, nausea, and sore throat.

Osteoarthritis

A gradual deterioration of the cartilage that lines the joints of the spine and the vertebrae themselves, causing back pain and stiffness. Cervical osteoarthritis affects the neck.

Prolapsed disk *(slipped disk)*

When one of the soft disks in between the spinal vertebrae (most often in the lower back) ruptures and bulges out onto a nerve root, intense pain results. It may be due to injury or gradual degeneration of the fibrous outer casing of the disk.

Sciatica

Intense pain along the sciatic nerve, which extends from the back of the thigh down to the calf of the leg. Sciatica is often caused by a slipped disk.

DIAGNOSIS AND TREATMENT

Diagnosis needs to be made by a doctor and may include physical examination, X-ray (to see joints and bones), MRI (magnetic resonance imaging, which allows soft tissue to be seen), CT scanning (computed tomagraphy, which shows the ligaments and blood supply as well as the skeleton), blood analysis, or other medical tests. Treatment varies according to the condition, but may include rest, painkillers, anti-inflammatories, heat treatment, massage, and supervised exercise.

INDEX

INDEX

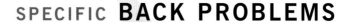

SPECIFIC **BACK PROBLEMS**

While much back pain is caused by strain or poor posture, it can also be

the result of a specific condition. The diagnosis of such back problems

must be made by a qualified medical practitioner, and self-help measures

should not be undertaken unless recommended by the practitioner.

Ankylosing spondylitis

Inflammation of the joints between the spinal vertebrae. Disks and ligaments calcify and "lock" together, making the spine increasingly stiff and sometimes hunched.

Coccydynia

Pain around the coccyx (tailbone), often caused by a fall.

Fibrositis

Pain and stiffness of the muscles, which may be caused by prolonged tension.

Infections

Kidney and viral infections, such as flu, can also cause back pain. Accompanying symptoms may include a temperature of 100°F (38°C) or above, diarrhea, nausea, and sore throat.

Osteoarthritis

A gradual deterioration of the cartilage that lines the joints of the spine and the vertebrae themselves, causing back pain and stiffness. Cervical osteoarthritis affects the neck.

Prolapsed disk *(slipped disk)*

When one of the soft disks in between the spinal vertebrae (most often in the lower back) ruptures and bulges out onto a nerve root, intense pain results. It may be due to injury or gradual degeneration of the fibrous outer casing of the disk.

Sciatica

Intense pain along the sciatic nerve, which extends from the back of the thigh down to the calf of the leg. Sciatica is often caused by a slipped disk.

DIAGNOSIS AND TREATMENT

Diagnosis needs to be made by a doctor and may include physical examination, X-ray (to see joints and bones), MRI (magnetic resonance imaging, which allows soft tissue to be seen), CT scanning (computed tomagraphy, which shows the ligaments and blood supply as well as the skeleton), blood analysis, or other medical tests. Treatment varies according to the condition, but may include rest, painkillers, anti-inflammatories, heat treatment, massage, and supervised exercise.

CREDITS

Quarto would like thank all those who took part in the special photography featured this book: Chrissie Dean (model), Geoff Burton (model), Deborah Doole (osteopath), and Georgiana Burrowcliff (acupuncturist).

We would also like to express our gratitude to Bushmaster Natural Health Practice for kindly allowing us to use its facilities for photography.

Bushmaster Natural Health Practice
204 Uxbridge Road
London W12 7JD
Tel: (UK) 0181 749 3792
Fax: (UK) 0181 749 0093

Quarto would like to acknowledge and thank the following for providing the pictures reproduced on the following pages of this book:

British Chiropractic Association pp94, 95
The Image Bank pp96, 97

All other photographs and illustrations are the copyright of Quarto.